The Source for Pediatric Dysphagia

Nancy B. Swigert

Skill Area: Dysphagia
Ages: Birth thru 18

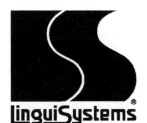

LinguiSystems, Inc.
3100 4th Avenue
East Moline, IL 61244-9700

800-776-4332

FAX: 800-577-4555
E-mail: service@linguisystems.com
Web: linguisystems.com

Copyright © 1998 LinguiSystems, Inc.

All of our products are copyrighted to protect the fine work of our authors. Copying this entire book for any reason is prohibited. You may, however, copy the worksheets as needed for your own use with students except for page 113, which may not be copied at any time.

Any other reproduction or distribution of these worksheets is not allowed, including copying this book to use as another primary source or "master" copy.

The enclosed CD is for your personal use and convenience. It is unlawful to copy this CD or store its content on a multi-user network.

Printed in the U.S.A.
ISBN 10: 0-7606-0236-0
ISBN 13: 978-0-7606-0236-2

About the Author

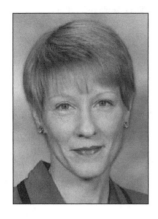

Nancy B. Swigert, M.A., CCC-SLP, received her master's degree from the University of Tennessee, Knoxville. She is the director and owner of Swigert & Associates, Inc., a private practice which has been providing services in the Lexington, KY area for over 18 years. The practice is contracted by Central Baptist Hospital in Lexington to run their Speech-Language Pathology Department. Nancy spends the majority of her time at the hospital as well as overseeing the provision of services in a variety of other settings including preschools, home health, and outpatient clinics.

In addition to administering her private practice and the speech-language department at the hospital, Nancy spends much of her time providing patient care. She evaluates and treats children and adults with dysphagia and with neurological communication disorders. Nancy lectures extensively at the state, regional, and national levels on dysphagia, dysarthria, and functional outcomes. She is also the author of *The Source for Dysphagia* and *The Source for Dysarthria*.

Nancy is the Past President of the Kentucky Speech-Language-Hearing Association and the Council of State Association Presidents. She is very active in the American Speech-Language-Hearing Association, serving as project officer for the Treatment Outcomes Project since its inception in 1994 and serving as ASHA President in 1998.

Acknowledgments

A private practice is successful, not based on the strength of one person in the practice, but based on the many varied talents of all those in the practice. I am lucky to have many fine pediatric clinicians as associates, and several have made significant contributions to this book:

> Verity Mathews, M.A., CCC-SLP, for capturing on paper her expertise with behavioral swallowing disorders in Chapter 8.
>
> Michelle Lankster, M.A., CCC-SLP, for contributing to our knowledge of infants' behavior related to breast feeding in Chapter 7.
>
> Janice Hensley, M.A., CCC-SLP, for sharing her knowledge of characteristics of premature babies.

We are also lucky to have a wonderful support staff who made sense of scribbled notes and rewrites and found missing references: Geri Cobb, Stephanie Castle, and June Ballman.

A special thanks to the following individuals at Central Baptist Hospital where we are fortunate to have the opportunity to practice:

> The nurses and physicians in the neonatal intensive care unit who allow us to participate in the care of their patients.
>
> Kathy Johnson, R.D., L.D., registered dietician who helps us understand the nutritional needs of these infants.
>
> Lonnie Wright and Jeff Kurz, librarians who can find just the right reference to round out our understanding of a topic.

Dedications

To the parents and caregivers of infants and children with dysphagia who work so diligently to help these children learn how to eat.

To Keith, for graciously understanding why I became so engrossed in writing this book, and for supporting my efforts.

Illustrations by Eulala Conner
Page Layout by Christine Buysse

Table of Contents

Introduction 7

Chapter 1: Anatomy and Physiology 9
Structures 9
Coordination of Sucking, Swallowing, and Breathing 14
Phases of Swallow 14
Suckling/Sucking 16
Normal Development of Feeding Skills 19
Normal Development of Self-feeding Skills 22
Appendix 1-A: Structural Differences in Suckling and Sucking 23
Appendix 1-B: Reflexes and What They Mean 24
References 25

Chapter 2: Medical Disorders 27
Premature Infants 27
Methods of Nutrition 30
Gastroesophageal Reflux Disease 32
Short Bowel Syndrome 35
AIDS 36
Cerebral Palsy 38
Head Injury 40
Fetal Alcohol Syndrome 43
Airway Feeding Problems 43
Congenital Heart Disease 48
Failure to Thrive 49
Craniofacial Anomalies 50
Pierre Robin and Micrognathia 53
Moëbius Sequence 55
References 56

Chapter 3: Clinical Evaluation of Infants & Children 61
Differences in Adults and Children 63
Instructions for Completing the *Infant Feeding Evaluation* 65
Example *Infant Feeding Evaluation* 78
Infant Feeding Evaluation 81
Example *Case History Form for Infants* 84
Case History Form for Infants 86
Instructions for Completing the *Pediatric Feeding Evaluation* . . . 88
Example *Pediatric Feeding Evaluation* 99
Pediatric Feeding Evaluation 102
Example *Case History Form for Children* 105
Case History Form for Children 109
Appendix 3-A: Interpretation of Feeding History 113
References 114

Chapter 4: Instrumentation, Devices, and Diagnostic Procedures 117
Modified Barium Swallow 117
Other Procedures 122
Monitors 123
Suctioning 124
Tube Feeding 124
Appendix 4-A: Barium Cookie Recipe 126
References 127

Chapter 5: Treatment of Feeding Disorders 128
Posture and Positioning 131
Oral-Motor Treatment 134
Specific Problems that Interfere with Feeding 135
Charts with Treatment Techniques 140
Description of Treatment Techniques 146
Food Presentation 154
References 159

Table of Contents, *continued*

Chapter 6: Treatment Techniques for Infants 161
   Distress Signals During Feeding ... 161
   Assessing State of Alertness 162
   Developing Oral-Motor and
      Suck-Swallow Skills 164
   Problems That Interfere with
      Adequate Suck 165
   Problems Associated with
      Coordinating Sucking,
      Swallowing, and Breathing 169
   Disorders in the Pharyngeal
      Stage of Swallowing 171
   References 173

Chapter 7: Breast-feeding and the Child with a Feeding Disorder 174
   Advantages/Disadvantages of
      Breast-feeding 174
   How Breast-feeding Works 174
   Readiness for Breast-feeding 176
   Problems That Can Occur
      with Breast-feeding 176
   Suggestions for Intervention 178
   Transition from Tube Feeding 180
   References 182

Chapter 8: Behavioral Feeding Problems 184
   Assessment 186
   Establishing a Plan of Treatment .. 188
   Behavioral-Based Intervention 188
   Techniques to Increase Behavior .. 190
   Techniques to Decrease Behavior . 191
   Skill Acquisition Techniques 193
   Other Therapeutic Approaches ... 194
   Other Considerations 195
   Behavioral Feeding Disorders
      and Families 197
   Working with Children Who Take
      Nothing by Mouth 198

   When an Inpatient Program
      Is Needed 202
   Example *Food Diary* 204
   Food Diary 205
   Example *Observation of
      Eating* 206
   Observation of Eating 207
   Appendix 8-A: Ways to Prevent
      or Minimize Feeding Problems ... 208
   Appendix 8-B: Information
      About Feeding Therapy 210
   References 212

Chapter 9: Drooling 216
   Anatomy and Physiology
      of Drooling 216
   Assessing Oral-Motor Function,
      Swallowing, and Drooling 218
   Options for Treatment 219
   Appendix 9-A: Questionnaire for
      Children with Severe Drooling ... 222
   References 223

Chapter 10: Goals and Treatment Objectives 224
   Long-Term Goals 225
   Short-Term Goals 226

Chapter 11: Tools for Feeding ... 240
   Seating Devices 241
   Pacifiers 242
   Nipples 243
   Bottles 244
   Cups 245
   Spoons 247
   Other Utensils and Tools 248
   References 249

Glossary 250

Introduction

Having authored *The Source for Dysphagia* two years ago, I eagerly agreed to write *The Source for Pediatric Dysphagia*. I did so because of my interest in dysphagia with patients of all ages, but also because I thought it would be easy to pull together this book having already done the first. However, writing this book served daily to remind me that treating infants and children with dysphagia is an entirely different task than treating adults. As clinicians, we would benefit from remembering that lesson (as would both our pediatric and adult patients)!

Infants and children present with different etiologies for their dysphagia, and many times do not present with a clearly defined etiology at all. Infants and children are constantly changing, as that's the nature of development, which means we are trying to hit a moving target. There are significant differences in the physiology and anatomy of the swallowing mechanism of the child and the adult. The adult can often describe the symptoms and tell us what is wrong. It is a rare occasion when the child can do so. Adults are often able to learn techniques to help with their swallowing, but with children, we have to perform more hands-on techniques.

The Source for Pediatric Dysphagia is designed to help clinicians who evaluate and treat infants and children with dysphagia organize their treatment approach. The information in this book will help you evaluate and treat a wide age range of children, from newborns through adolescents with developmental disabilities, including cerebral palsy. As with any discussion of a disorder, we must begin with a reminder of what is normal. Understanding how typical infants and children develop their swallowing skills helps us develop treatment programs that make sense developmentally.

This book provides you with practical tips on how to evaluate infants and children, including two different case history and evaluation forms. One is for young infants and the other for children over four months of age. These forms should help you record your observations of the child's ability to eat and drink, as well as your observations of how the caregiver interacts with the child. The book describes treatment techniques that you will use with many children, and includes a separate chapter on techniques especially designed for infants.

The Source for Pediatric Dysphagia should also help you reduce the amount of time you spend on paperwork. Chapter 10 has long- and short-term goals and treatment objectives organized by the type of oral-motor or behavioral problem you are addressing. These goals will keep you from reinventing the wheel for each child you see, yet will allow you to customize the goals to meet a specific child's needs.

There are so many things to remember and consider when working with infants and children with dysphagia. I hope *The Source for Pediatric Dysphagia* helps you refine your skills and organize your approach to treatment.

Nancy

Chapter 1: Anatomy and Physiology

Any guide to the evaluation and treatment of a disorder must begin with an understanding of the anatomy, physiology, and normal development of the process.

The relationship between sucking, swallowing, and breathing is a critical one to understand as this is one of the main ways that pediatric swallowing differs from swallowing disorders in adults. These three processes are very interrelated because the structures for these three functions are very close together and they share neurologic innervation. Because of the relationship of the processes, the structures of the upper and lower aerodigestive tracts must be understood. The upper aerodigestive tract consists of the nasal and oral cavities, pharynx, larynx, trachea, and esophagus. The lower airway consists of the lungs. The lower digestive tract is the stomach and small and large intestines.

Structures

Nasal Cavity The nasal cavity warms and cleans air before it enters the lungs. The nasal cavity is separated from the oral cavity by the hard palate and soft palate.

Oral Cavity The oral cavity (i.e., mouth) plays an important role in eating, vocalizing, and breathing. The major structures of the oral cavity include the following:

- lips
- mandible
- maxilla
- floor of the mouth
- cheeks
- tongue
- hard palate
- soft palate
- anterior and posterior faucial arches
- teeth (in older children)

Although it's not actually a structure, it is also important to pay attention to the anterior and lateral sulci (i.e., the spaces between the mandible or maxilla and the cheeks or lips).

Pharynx The pharynx is crucial in both swallowing and respiration. It is comprised of three parts:

Nasopharynx The nasopharynx does not have much of a role in the act of swallowing. In fact, it should be closed off by the soft palate during swallowing. If there is any velopharyngeal incompetence, there may be some nasal reflux or back flow into the nasopharynx, especially with liquids. The adenoids are on the back wall of the nasopharynx. The only

Chapter 1: Anatomy and Physiology, *continued*

relationship they have to swallowing is that if they are very enlarged, they can stop an infant from breathing adequately through his nose and can sometimes interfere with feeding.

Oropharynx The oropharynx begins with the tonsillar pillars and extends to the posterior pharyngeal wall. The top boundary of the oropharynx is the lower surface of the soft palate. The oropharynx also extends to the base of tongue, the hyoid bone, and the tip of the epiglottis.

Hypopharynx The hypopharynx extends from the tip of the epiglottis down to the cricopharyngeus muscle. It also is the inlet to the larynx down to the level of the false cords.

Larynx The larynx serves three primary functions:

- protects the airway
- aids in respiration
- aids in phonation

Movement of the larynx and, internally, the true and false vocal cords, is responsible for achieving airway closure during swallowing. The hyoid and larynx lift up and forward while the epiglottis is pushed down. The arytenoid cartilages tilt forward and the false and true cords close. All of these mechanisms work together to close off the airway for protection during swallowing.

Trachea The trachea is comprised of *C*-shaped cartilaginous rings. A soft membrane makes up the posterior part of the trachea and the anterior wall of the esophagus. This is a common wall.

Esophagus The esophagus is a muscular tube that remains closed until food travels through it. The cricopharyngeus or upper esophageal sphincter serves as the junction between the hypopharynx and the esophagus. The lower esophageal sphincter is the junction between the esophagus and the stomach.

Chapter 1: Anatomy and Physiology, *continued*

It is the job of these two sphincters to keep the esophagus empty between swallows. The upper esophageal sphincter's job is to keep air from entering the esophagus from above and the lower esophageal sphincter's job is to keep food from coming up from the stomach.

The upper third of the esophagus is comprised of striated muscle similar to the pharynx, while the lower two-thirds is a smooth muscle fiber. The pharynx and upper third of the esophagus are the only regions in the body where striated muscle is not under voluntary neural control (Arvedson, Rogers, and Brodsky, 1993). They are innervated by both sympathetic and parasympathetic fibers.

Recurrent laryngeal nerves travel on either side of the esophagus. Other structures related to breathing and feeding that are close to the esophagus include the left main stem bronchus, the aortic arch, the pericardium, and esophageal nerves and blood vessels.

Several distinctive differences exist between pediatric and adult anatomy. In a newborn, the connection between the nasopharynx and the hypopharynx is a gentle curve. In an adult, there is almost a 90° angle between the nasopharynx and the hypopharynx.

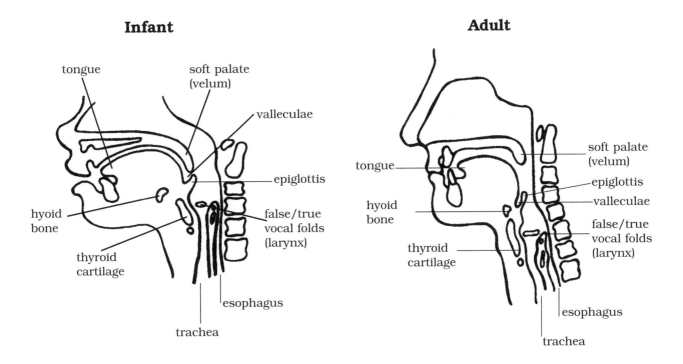

Chapter 1: Anatomy and Physiology, *continued*

The base of the tongue and the larynx descend during the first four years of life. Caruso and Sauerland (1990) indicate that by age four, the base of the tongue has descended far enough that it actually forms the anterior wall of the oropharynx. These changes continue during childhood and accelerate during puberty.

Infants have sucking pads (i.e., fatty tissues in the cheeks). These sucking pads usually disappear between four to six months of age.

An infant's tongue fills his mouth and sits more anteriorly than an adult's. The mandible is smaller, which makes the tongue seem oversized.

The tongue, soft palate, pharynx, and larynx, which are higher in the neck of an infant, facilitate nasal breathing during swallowing. This continues through the first 3-4 months of life when most infants typically start to breathe through their mouths as well as their noses (Arvedson et al., 1993). The chart on page 13 describes the structural differences between infants and older children.

Chapter 1: Anatomy and Physiology, *continued*

Structural Differences Between Infants and Older Children

Infants	Older Children
Stability is provided positionally (i.e., various structures are very close to one another and the infant has a large amount of subcutaneous fat).	Stability is provided posturally with the structures moving farther apart as the child grows. Then the child relies on connective tissue and more highly specialized muscle control to provide stability for swallowing.
The tongue fills almost the entire oral cavity—touching cheeks, hard palate, and soft palate.	With growth, the tongue drops down and moves posteriorly in the mouth. This opens up space to allow for chewing motion and also allows the child to have room for more tongue movements.
Tongue tip sticks out past the alveolar ridge and touches the lower lip.	Tongue tip is behind alveolar ridge.
The fat pads (sucking pads) in the cheeks help support oral and pharyngeal function (Bosma, 1972).	As fat pads disappear, stability of the mandible is provided by more muscle control. As the cheeks become less fat, the child is able to obtain more movement of the lips and cheeks.
The soft palate is large. The uvula is close to the tip of the epiglottis.	As the child grows and the pharynx elongates, the soft palate moves away from the epiglottis. At that point, the base of the tongue becomes a more important structure in swallowing.
Faucial arches touch the epiglottis on either side. This may allow for accumulation of the bolus in the valleculae during consecutive sucking.	Faucial arches do not touch the epiglottis.
The hyoid and larynx are very close together and very near the mandible, much higher in the neck than in an older child.	The hyoid and larynx move farther apart. Each begins to demonstrate more mobility.
The shape of the opening to the larynx is affected by muscle action. It is possible that infants may show more penetration than older children.	Entrance to airway more tightly closed.

Chapter 1: Anatomy and Physiology, *continued*

Coordination of Sucking, Swallowing, and Breathing

Relationship Between Breathing and Swallowing

Infants prefer to breathe through their noses because of the anatomy. When an infant initiates a swallow, the bolus moves over the back of the tongue and the mechanisms for airway protection initiate. That is, the true and false cords close and the larynx pulls up and forward with epiglottis and aryepiglottic folds bunching together to close off the top entrance to the airway.

It had been thought that infants did not have to coordinate breathing and swallowing. It was believed that because of their anatomy, infants could continue to breathe when swallowing because liquid was swallowed safely on either side of the larynx. However, Wilson et al. (1980) showed that a swallow always coincided with cessation of nasal airflow. That is, infants stopped breathing briefly with every swallow. The cessation in breathing lasted about one second. This was confirmed by Weber (1986) who indicated that infants stopped breathing when swallowing.

There does not seem to be an agreement about when in the respiratory cycle the infant stops breathing. Some studies have shown it to be after expiration. Others have shown it to be after inspiration. It is known that during continuous sucking, infants have a decrease in their overall respiratory rate. They also lengthen their expiratory phase and shorten their inspiratory phase. This leads to a reduction in minute ventilation (i.e., the amount of air breathed in one minute).

Some authors (Shivpuri et al., 1983) hypothesize that the stopping of breathing during continuous sucking leads to a change in blood chemistry, which then triggers the infant to change to an intermittent sucking pattern.

The swallowing pattern is related to the flow and amount of liquid. If an infant sucks at a faster rate, he will have to swallow more often. If an infant sucks with greater pressure, more bolus will enter his mouth and the infant may have to adjust his timing for initiating swallowing.

Phases of Swallow

There are four phases of the swallow: oral preparatory, oral (voluntary), pharyngeal, and esophageal. The oral preparatory and oral (voluntary) phases are entirely voluntary. The pharyngeal phase has a voluntary and involuntary component. The esophageal phase is completely involuntary.

During the **oral preparatory phase**, the child manipulates food or liquid in the mouth to form it into a bolus. In infants, this is when sucking occurs. In older children who are eating foods that have to be chewed, the oral preparatory phase takes longer. What happens during this phase?

Chapter 1: Anatomy and Physiology, *continued*

- Lips close around nipple or cup so no liquid is lost out the front of the mouth.

- Liquid is moved around in the mouth and a bolus is formed.

- The bolus is held between the tongue and hard palate.

- The soft palate is pulled forward against the base of the tongue to keep the bolus from falling into the pharynx.

- The airway is open and nasal breathing continues.

The **oral (voluntary) phase** begins as soon as the child starts propelling the bolus posteriorly. It ends when the bolus has left the oral cavity. Because the bolus is already formed and is resting on top of the tongue before this phase begins, the timing of this phase does not vary according to texture. It typically takes less than one second for an infant with normal development to push any bolus over the back of his tongue. What happens during this phase?

- The tongue is elevated toward the soft palate.

- The tongue presses against the roof of the mouth in a peristaltic motion to squeeze the food or liquid backward (Ramsey et al., 1955).

- The soft palate elevates and closes off the nasopharynx.

- The bolus leaves the mouth.

The **pharyngeal phase** begins with the initiation of the pharyngeal swallow. What happens during this phase?

- The true vocal folds close as the arytenoid cartilages come together.

- The false vocal folds close.

- The arytenoid cartilages tip forward to touch the base of the epiglottis.

- The hyoid and larynx are pulled up and forward.

- The epiglottis is pushed down to deflect the bolus to either side and to move it posteriorly away from the airway (Shaker et al., 1990).

- The bolus is propelled through the pharynx by pressure created by the base of the tongue, some movement of the pharyngeal walls, and the opening of the upper esophageal sphincter (caused by lifting the larynx). As the bolus moves through the pharynx, it divides so that approximately half moves through a pyriform sinus at each side of the pharynx. Then the bolus rejoins right above the level of the upper esophageal sphincter (Ardran and Kemp, 1951).

Chapter 1: Anatomy and Physiology, continued

It appears that the pharyngeal phase occurs from the bottom up, with closure of the true vocal folds occurring first. Other studies have indicated that the false vocal folds also close during swallowing (Sasaki and Isaacson, 1988).

During the **esophageal phase**, a peristaltic wave helps move the bolus through the esophagus and into the stomach. If there is a delay between distinctly different pharyngeal swallows, an esophageal peristaltic wave will be observed for each pharyngeal swallow. The esophageal phase in infants may not be observed until after four or more pharyngeal swallows, or it may even be delayed until the end of an active burst of suckling (Arvedson et al., 1993; Bosma, 1986). An infant often swallows air along with the milk, and therefore needs to be burped.

Suckling/Sucking

Infants begin the swallowing process with a suckle. Sometime between six and nine months of age, an infant moves from a suckle pattern to a true suck. There are significant differences in the actions of the oral structures during suckling and sucking. These differences are highlighted in Appendix 1-A on page 23.

They engage in nutritive and non-nutritive suckling. According to Wolf and Glass (1992), there are some differences in the patterns observed. (See the chart below.)

Nutritive Suckling	**Non-nutritive Suckling**
At the beginning of a feeding, an infant sucks with a continuous burst and then changes to more intermittent bursts of sucking. The bursts become shorter, with longer pauses in between as the feeding proceeds.	The pattern is much more repetitive than with nutritive sucking.
One suck per second	Six sucks per second
Young infants swallow with a one-to-one ratio to their sucking (i.e., for every suck, they swallow). This is necessary because every time they pull liquid into their mouths, they have to swallow it. They may suck a few more times before a swallow near the end of a feeding. As the infant becomes older (several months), the ratio may be two or three sucks to one swallow. This may be because the oral cavity is larger and child can hold more in the oral cavity.	Six or eight sucks per swallow

The Source for Pediatric Dysphagia

Chapter 1: Anatomy and Physiology, *continued*

When an infant's lips close around a nipple, they turn partially outward (i.e., the inner part of the lips touches the nipple). It is normal for a young infant to fail to get a tight approximation around the nipple which may cause some milk to leak at either side of the nipple.

Infants with normal development often have a hard time getting started on a regular suckling pattern. They may not start with good compressions against the nipple. They may have some gasping or choking because they don't have the oral cavity tightly sealed from the pharynx. However, a typical infant will then move into a more rhythmic pattern of suckle feeding. When gasping or choking happens, the infant appears able to bring the material not ready to be swallowed back into the mouth from the pharynx. Bosma (1986) terms this "normal choking" or "pharyngeal regurgitation."

Both positive and negative pressure are used to expel milk from the nipple. Positive pressure occurs when fluid is compressed, squeezed, or pushed out of something (e.g., squeezing a tube of toothpaste to press the toothpaste out of the tube). Negative pressure is similar to a suction action (e.g., using a syringe to draw fluid up from a cup). Negative pressure or suction is created when there is a change in the pressure gradient and the fluid wants to flow into the area of less pressure.

During a suckle, the tongue, lower lip, mandible, and hyoid move together as a single entity. The tongue, lip, mandible, and hyoid move down and forward and then up and back. The down-and-forward movement causes the negative pressure. The up-and-back movement causes the compression. This down-and-forward and up-and-back movement during suckling occurs about two times per second. It may be slower if the nipple is larger (Bosma, 1986).

During sucking, the front of the infant's tongue pushes against the nipple and causes positive pressure. The back of the infant's tongue lowers (as does the jaw a little bit) to increase the volume of the oral cavity which creates the negative pressure or suction.

Factors affecting the amount of pressure generated during sucking

More Pressure	**Less Pressure**
• awake/alert	• sleepy
• hungry	• full
• sweet liquid	• non-sweet liquid
• slow fluid flow	• fast fluid flow

Chapter 1: Anatomy and Physiology, continued

In infant feeding, both positive and negative pressure are important, though more pressure can be generated from negative than positive pressure. With breast-feeding, negative pressure and suction are very important to draw the nipple into the infant's mouth and to keep it in position within the mouth. This is not so with a bottle, as a rigid nipple can be put into an infant's mouth with no suction needed to draw it in.

Sometime between six and nine months of age, an infant moves from a suckle pattern to a true suck. There are significant differences in the actions of the oral structures during suckling and sucking. These differences are highlighted in Apendix 1-A on page 23.

Infant's Response to Stimuli

When working with infants, it's important to understand the relationship between things that happen to the infant and the infant's response. The infant has many reflexes and responses that serve to protect the airway. These reflexes are triggered from receptors in the nose, nasopharynx, upper airway, and lungs. The reflexes can be triggered either by chemical receptors or mechanical receptors. Chemical receptors are those which respond to chemicals such as water, milk, secretions, acid, etc. Mechanical receptors respond to touch or pressure.

Any time an infant has a pause in respiration that is initiated by any of these receptors, it is considered apnea even if it is only for a short duration. A brief period of apnea can be protective because it closes the larynx and shuts the airway. If it continues, however, it could lead to hypoxia and possibly even bradycardia.

Normal Reflexes Observed

In typical infants who are ready to be fed, touching the area around the mouth should elicit rooting. This is the response of the head, neck, lips, and face to get into position for sucking. The mouth moves toward the nipple or similar object. This can usually be elicited with touches on the cheek, upper lip, or lower lip. The infant will start to root and continue until he latches on (Bosma, 1986).

In addition to the rooting reflex, several other reflexes are important for the development of early feeding skills. Suckling may not truly be reflexive, but when a nipple is placed in an infant's mouth or the top of an infant's tongue is stroked, the infant will begin a suckle movement. This reflex allows the infant to take liquid into his mouth.

Swallowing is also part reflexive in response to a bolus of food entering the pharynx. This reflex allows food to move from the pharynx into the esophagus. The tongue protrusion reflex is elicited by touching the front of the tongue. It is probably related to suckling which infants use for early bottle and breast-feeding. When it begins to disappear between four and six months of age, solids can be introduced on a spoon. Until that time, the tongue protrusion is counterproductive for introducing spoon eating.

Chapter 1: Anatomy and Physiology, continued

A phasic bite reflex is elicited with pressure to the gums and is responsible for early munching patterns. The gag reflex appears to have no relationship to swallowing in adults, but in infants, it begins to diminish in strength at around six months of age when solid foods are usually introduced.

These reflexes and their relationships to swallowing are summarized in Appendix 1-B on page 24.

Normal Development of Feeding Skills

Infants basically receive all of their nourishment through nipple feedings for the first four to six months of life. At that stage, transitional feeding begins. The change from nipple feeding to transitional feeding is related to central nervous system maturation more than any changes in the characteristics of the face and mouth (Bosma, 1986).

At four to six months of age, spoon feeding can usually be introduced. About one month later, cup drinking can be introduced. Illingsworth and Lister (1964) suggest that there appears to be a "critical and/or sensitive" period for introducing chewable textures to children. If solids are not introduced during this critical time, an important developmental milestone may be missed. This can lead to rejection of solid foods when they are introduced later. Children who are developing as expected should be able to chew foods at about six months of age.

Biting and Chewing

Initially, babies suck on food. By five to six months, they munch up and down, but they still can't bite through a cookie because they can't stabilize or hold the cookie in their teeth. At about nine months of age, they are able to hold a cookie between their teeth or gums while an adult breaks off a piece for them to chew. Between one and two years, you may see overflow movements during biting such as facial grimaces, twisting of the hands, or pulling back of the head. These movements indicate stress or that the food is too difficult to bite through. By age two, children can bite through most foods without overflow movements.

For a child to move toward taking food from a spoon and eating more solid foods, the child has to be able to close his lips around a spoon, use his incisors to bite, use other teeth to chew, use his tongue to form a bolus, and use his tongue to push the bolus back. Before a child has teeth, he "chews" by bringing the mandible and maxilla together. He protrudes the mandible forward from its typical resting position (Bosma, 1986).

As children begin eating more solid foods, they have to be able to move the food toward the side of the tongue and onto the chewing surface. Initially the child chews simply by opening and closing the mandible. It is not until later that a rotary chew involving lateral motion is developed.

The Source for Pediatric Dysphagia

Chapter 1: Anatomy and Physiology, *continued*

Pridom (1990) describes four basic stages of the development of feeding: taking food from a spoon, chewing, self-feeding, and managing cup or bottle. These steps develop between six and twelve months of age. The chart below and on the next page describes the steps and reflects the development of a child's abilities to communicate when full.

The ability to self-feed depends on the development of related gross and fine motor skills. The chart on page 22 delineates some of those relationships (Bosma, 1972).

Age in Months	Taking Food from a Spoon	Chewing	Self-feeding	Managing Cup or Bottle	Communicating Hunger/Satiety
5-7	takes semi-solid food from a spoon				
6		munching pattern using up and down motion; infant gums thicker food with small lumps			
6-7					infant may make sputtering noises or shake head when full
6-8				tongue protrusion continues with milk leaking from the corner of the mouth	
7-8				one to two swallows taken from a cup held by an adult; chokes easily	infant vocalizes eagerness when put in high chair or when sees feeding utensils
7-12		rotary chew may begin to develop			

continued

The Source for Pediatric Dysphagia

Chapter 1: Anatomy and Physiology, continued

Age in Months	Taking Food from a Spoon	Chewing	Self-feeding	Managing Cup or Bottle	Communicating Hunger/Satiety
8	quickly and efficiently removes food from a spoon using upper and lower lips and bringing head forward to accept the spoon	lateral movement of the tongue noted		holds bottle and tips it up	
9			reaches for spoon		
9-10				brings bottle to mouth; drinks from a cup that is held for him	
10		definite chewing movement			
10-11			good pincer grasp; usually prefers to finger feed than to be spoon fed		infant vocalizes impatient fussing if parent is slow presenting food; pivots away from feeder or throws food when full
12		takes controlled bites of soft foods or readily dissolved crunchy foods*	grasps spoon handle but doesn't handle spoon well	holds cup with two hands and takes 4-5 swallows continuously without choking	

* It appears that the coordination of chewing is fully mature by three to six years of age. (Vitti & Basmajian, 1975).

Chapter 1: Anatomy and Physiology, continued

Normal Development of Self-feeding Skills

Age in Months	Self-feeding Skills	Related Motor Development
0.5	hand to mouth begins	
2-4	hand on bottle during feeding	initiation of midline orientation of head, eyes, and hands
4	spoon feeding introduced	
4-6	cup drinking introduced	
5-6	both hands on bottle	
5-7	semi-solids from spoon	reaches for objects; reduction in anterior-posterior tongue action in suckling; able to sit without support
6	cracker to mouth briefly	
6	lip closure around spoon	
6	munching begins; vertical jaw action	spurt in gross motor development
7	chewing begins; rotary action	increased ability to move tongue laterally; ability to maintain bolus over the molars using lip closure and cheek action
6-8	liquids sucked from cup	
8-9	assists with spoon	able to bring head foward and use upper and lower lips together on spoon; head movements supported by trunk control
9	cracker to mouth; deliberately reaches for spoon	
9-10	drinks from cup held by caregiver	ability to sit without support gives mobility to shoulders and arms
10-11	pincer grasp for finger feeding	improves fine control of upper extremity and hand movements
12	self-feeds by grasping spoon with whole hand	
12	holds cup with two hands; 4-5 consecutive swallows	
12	holds and tips bottle by self	
15-24	skills refined for independent self-feeding	

The Source for Pediatric Dysphagia

Chapter 1: Anatomy and Physiology, continued

Appendix 1-A

Structural Differences in Suckling and Sucking

Oral Structure	What happens in suckling? (Birth to 6-9 months)	What happens in sucking? (Begins around 6-9 months)
tongue	backward and forward motion of the tongue tongue does not protrude past border of lips front of tongue (with the lips) seals against the nipple — the back of the tongue seals against the soft palate to keep liquid in the mouth until child is ready to swallow tongue is flat, thin, cupped, or bowl shaped	tongue body raises and lowers there is more room for tongue movement because oral cavity has grown down and forward tongue is flat, thin, slightly cupped, or bowl shaped
jaw	moves up and down	moves up and down less, but this still helps produce suction (i.e., negative pressure)
lips	loose approximation on nipple	tight approximation on nipple helps seal the nipple and stabilize the nipple in the mouth
cheeks	fat pads provide stability in the cheeks and keep food from accumulating in buccal cavities	continue to provide stability provide boundary on either side of tongue to keep liquid on tongue
hard palate	tongue presses against palate during forward and back motion	tongue presses against palate to create positive pressure on the nipple
soft palate	seals against back of tongue to keep liquid in mouth — may even move toward tongue lifts during swallowing to seal the nasopharynx to prevent liquid from entering the nasal cavity	same as in suckling except soft palate is not seen to move toward tongue

The Source for Pediatric Dysphagia

Chapter 1: Anatomy and Physiology, *continued*

Appendix 1-B

Reflexes and What They Mean

Reflex	How to Stimulate	Cranial Nerves	When does it disappear?	What does it mean for swallowing?
gag	touch posterior tongue or pharnyx	IX, X	remains in adults, though 30% of adults don't have one — does diminish at 6 months of age	no relationship; diminishes at 6 months of age, about the time chewing solids occurs
phasic bite	apply pressure to gums	V	9-12 months	allows early munching patterns
tongue protrusion	touch the front of the tongue	XII	4-6 months	can begin to introduce solids on a spoon when reflex disappears
rooting	touch corner of mouth	V, VII, XI, XII	3-6 months	helps the infant find the nipple
suckling (may not be purely reflexive)	put nipple in mouth or stroke top of tongue	V, VII, IX, XII	6-12 months	allows infants to take liquid into the mouth; when it diminishes, it allows the child to move towards cup drinking and eating from a spoon
swallowing	bolus of food in pharynx	V, VII, IX, X, XII	remains in adults	allows food to travel safely through pharynx to the esophagus

The Source for Pediatric Dysphagia

Chapter 1: Anatomy and Physiology, continued

References

Ardran, G.M. et al. "A Cineradiographic Study of Breast-feeding." *British Journal of Radiology*, Vol. 31, 1958, pp. 11-22, 156-162.

Ardran, G.M. and Kemp, F. "The Mechanism of Swallowing." *Proceedings of the Royal Society of Medicine*, Vol. 44, 1951, pp. 1038-1040.

Arvedson, J. et al. "Anatomy, Embryology, and Physiology." In Arvedson, J. and Brodsky, L. (eds.) *Pediatric Swallowing and Feeding: Assessment and Management*, San Diego: Singular Publishing Group, Inc., 1993, pp. 5-12.

Bosma, J.F. "Development of Feeding." *Clinical Nutrition*, Vol. 5, 1986, pp. 210-218.

Bosma, J.F. "Form and Function in the Infant's Mouth and Pharynx." In Bosma, J.F. (ed.) *Oral Sensation and Perception: The Mouth of the Infant*, Springfield, IL: Charles C. Thomas, 1972, pp. 3-29.

Bosma, J.F. "Functional Anatomy of the Upper Airway During Development." *Respiratory Function of the Upper Airway*, New York: Marcel Dekker, Inc., 1988, pp. 47-86.

Caruso, V.G. and Sauerland, E.K. "Embryology and Anatomy." In Bluestone, B.C. et al. *Pediatric Otolaryngology*, 2nd ed. Philadelphia: W. B. Saunders, Vol. 2, 1990, pp. 807-815.

Dodds, W.J. "The Physiology of Swallowing." *Dysphagia*, Vol. 3, 1989, pp. 171-178.

Dodds, W.J. et al. "Physiology and Radiology of the Normal Oral and Pharyngeal Phases of Swallowing." *American Journal of Radiology*, Vol. 154, 1990, pp. 953-963.

Ekberg, O. "Closure of the Laryngeal Vestibule During Deglutition." *ACTA Otolarygologica*, Vol. 93, 1982, pp. 123-129.

Illingsworth, R.S. and Lister, J. "The Critical or Sensitive Period, with Special Reference to Certain Feeding Problems in Infants and Children." *The Journal of Pediatrics*, Vol. 65, 1964, pp. 839-848.

Miller, A.J. "Neurophysiologic Basis of Swallowing." *Dysphagia*, Vol. 1, 1986, pp. 91-100.

Pridom, K.F. "Feeding Behavior of 6 - 12 Month Old Infants: Assessment and Sources of Parental Information." *The Journal of Pediatrics*, Vol. 117, 1990, pp. 174-180.

Ramsey, G.H. et al. "Cinefluorographic Analysis of the Mechanism of Swallowing." *Radiology*, Vol. 64, 1955, pp. 498-518.

Sasaki, C.T. and Isaacson, G. "Functional Anatomy of the Larynx." *Otolaryngology Clinics of North America*, Vol. 21, 1988, pp. 196-199.

Shaker, R. et al. "Coordination of Deglutitive Glottic Closure with Oropharyngeal Swallowing." *Gastroenterology*, Vol. 98, 1990, pp. 1478-1484.

Chapter 1: Anatomy and Physiology, continued

Shivpuri, C.R. et al. "Decreased Ventilation in Preterm Infants During Oral Feeding." *The Journal of Pediatrics*, Vol. 103, 1983, pp. 285-289.

Smith, W.L. et al. "Imaging Evaluation of the Human Nipple During Breast-Feeding." *American Journal of Diseases in Children*, Vol. 142, 1988, pp. 76-78.

Tuchman, D.N. and Walter, R.S. *Disorders of Feeding and Swallowing in Infants and Children — Pathophysiology, Diagnosis, and Treatment.* San Diego: Singular Publishing Group, Inc., 1994.

Vitti, M. and Basmajian, J.V. "Muscles of Mastication in Small Children: An Electromyographic Analysis." *American Journal of Orthodontics*, Vol. 68, 1975, pp. 412-419.

Weber, F.M. et al. "An Ultrasonographic Study of the Organization of Sucking and Swallowing by Newborn Infants." *Developmental Medicine and Child Neurology*, Vol. 28, 1986, pp. 19-24.

Wilson, S.L. et al. "Upper Airway Patency in the Human Infant: Influence of Airway Pressure and Posture." *Journal of Applied Physiology*, Vol. 48, 1980, pp. 500-504.

Wolf, L.F. and Glass, R.P. *Feeding and Swallowing Disorders in Infancy: Assessment and Management.* San Antonio: Therapy Skill Builders, a division of The Psychological Corporation, 1992.

Chapter 2: Medical Disorders

This chapter includes descriptions of specific medical problems that may result in dysphagia. Many of the problems described in this chapter are treated with the same oral-motor techniques as described in Chapter 5. However, there are specific treatments suggested in this chapter for dysphagia associated with the disorders described. For instance, there is an extensive description of feeding disorders in children with cleft lip and palate. Treatment techniques are included here rather than in the treatment chapter.

This chapter is not meant to be all inclusive of every kind of medical disorder that can have a related pediatric dysphagia. Instead, it contains information about commonly occurring problems, or those problems which have a more significant impact on feeding. Information is provided about the medical disorder and medical/surgical treatment, as well as information about the impact the medical disorder has on the child's ability to eat.

Premature Infants

An infant is considered premature if the gestational period is less than 36 weeks. The complications resulting from premature births vary from minimal amounts of medical attention necessary to very medically fragile. Premature infants frequently are not capable of oral feeding due to poorly organized sucking bursts, disorganized jaw and tongue movement, immature lungs which make them intolerant of apneic periods during swallowing, and other neurological and circulatory immaturity.

Numerous reports indicate that pre-term infants with very low birth weight (VLBW) and chronic illnesses are at increased risk for feeding disorders that can negatively affect growth and development. It is also recognized that the parents' response to infant feeding disorders, including anxiety exhibited by the mother, can contribute to feeding disorders. Several studies have analyzed maternal/infant interaction and most find that the interaction between mothers and pre-term infants is different from the interaction between mothers and their full-term or healthier counterparts. Pre-term infants are less responsive, less interactive, and fussier with less positive affect and fewer vocalizations than their full-term peers in both feeding and play situations with their mothers. Mothers' reactions to pre-term infants have also been found to be different than their reactions to full-term babies. This is not surprising given that many infants with VLBW have chronic illnesses which require a significantly higher level of caregiving than do healthy children.

Although the fetus has been observed through ultrasound swallowing amniotic fluid as early as 13 weeks, the premature infant is unable to coordinate sucking, swallowing, and breathing until 34 weeks gestational age (Shaker, 1990). Therefore, many professionals do not begin feeding premature infants before age 34-35 weeks (Agnos, 1998; Shaker, 1990), although successful feeding of infants can occur as early as 30-31 weeks of gestation (Agnos, 1998). When determining if

Chapter 2: Medical Disorders, continued

the infant is ready to begin eating, Wolf et al. (1992) note that "maturation as measured by gestational age is the key to readiness opposed to weight or chronological age."

The oral cavity of a premature infant also puts her at a disadvantage for feeding. The premature infant does not have sucking pads. Sucking pads decrease the size of the oral cavity, provide positional stability, and facilitate the compression between the cheek and tongue.

Special Diagnostic Categories Related to Prematurity

Intercranial Hemorrhage (ICH) is a frequent complication of prematurity. Wolf et al. (1992) stated ICH occurs in one-third to one-half of infants weighing less than 1500 grams, usually noted in the neonatal period. ICH results in bleeding in the brain which leads to numerous complications including gross motor disorders, visual deficits, speech delays, and swallowing disorders. The type of injury depends on the location and extent of hemorrhagic damage.

Necrotizing Enterocolitis (NEC) is a gastrointestinal disease which is most commonly seen in premature infants, but may also be seen in full-term infants. NEC produces excessive gas which causes or adds to mucosal injury in the esophagus and can lead to a perforated bowel (Agnos, 1998). If the bowel becomes perforated, the infant will require surgery. Surgery can lead to short gut syndrome (i.e., Short Bowel Syndrome) if enough of the bowel is removed.

NEC usually develops within three to ten days of life (Wolf and Glass, 1992). Diagnostic signs of NEC include feeding intolerance (i.e., emesis), abdominal distention, and gastric retention of feedings (Agnos, 1998; Wolf and Glass, 1992). Premature infants with NEC are often NPO (i.e., no gavage feedings) and receive total parenteral nutrition (TPN). The infant is placed on "bowel rest," receives antibiotics, and has surgery if needed. Intake by mouth is slowly introduced. There are frequent setbacks.

Infant Respiratory Distress Syndrome (IRDS) is common in infants born before 35-36 weeks due to immature lungs and the inability to produce sufficient amounts of surfactant (i.e., a substance in the lungs which helps keep the alveoli inflated). More than 70% of infants less than 28 weeks gestation develop IRDS. There is an inadequate amount of surfactant in the alveoli which leads to respiratory insufficiency (Wolf and Glass, 1992).

Bronchopulmonary Dysplasia (BPD) is frequently seen in neonates who have received positive pressure ventilation. Most infants with BPD had IRDS and did not fully recover from the IRDS. Infants with BPD have an increased respiratory effort, increased respiratory rates, decreased pulmonary compliance, impaired gas exchange, and increased respiratory fatigue (Agnos, 1998).

Chapter 2: Medical Disorders, continued

Infants weighing under 1000 grams develop BPD 50-85% of the time, whereas premature infants weighing over 1000 grams develop BPD only 5-16% of the time. The increased incidence of BPD with lower birth weight is probably related to immature lungs (Bancalari, 1986).

BPD is generally treated with oxygen, steroids, and diuretics (Agnos, 1998). BPD increases the difficulty of feeding because the infant cannot regulate breathing and swallowing, has decreased endurance, and is usually more orally defensive. During feedings, it is important to pace the infant, provide frequent breaks, burp frequently, and increase the amount of oxygen.

Congenital Heart Disease is caused by a deficit in the cardiovascular system and results in abnormal blood flow. Premature infants have increased heart rates and blood pressure because they are trying to compensate for their inability to pump enough blood (Agnos, 1998). Feeding is difficult for infants with congenital heart disease because of increased oxygen demands during feedings. To increase success with feedings, use more external support, provide frequent breaks, and use higher caloric formula. Because of the infant's weak suck and lack of endurance, a high flow or soft nipple should be used. Proceed with extreme caution to avoid overwhelming the infant with too much flow of formula.

Reflexes Related to Feeding

There are several reflexes necessary for successful feeding in the premature infant, although some of these reflexes are not present until the infant becomes closer to the age of a full-term baby.

Gestational Age in Weeks	Reflex
23-24	brief periods of an arrhythmical sucking reflex, but not a swallowing reflex
25-26	rooting reflex beginning to emerge; sucking reflex continues to improve
27-28	beginning of the swallow reflex, although it is not complete[1]
30	rooting reflex continues to improve; suck-swallow reflex occurs more regularly
32	improved coordination of swallowing; active and strong sucking reflex; rooting reflex is complete
33	Santmyer Swallow reflex[2]
34-35	coordination and strength to begin bottle feeding
37	suck-swallow reflex like that of a full-term infant[3]

[1] An infant at 28 weeks improves rhythm with sucking, but tires easily (Morris, 1987).

[2] The Santmyer Swallow is elicited by gently blowing in the infant's face. The infant should respond by swallowing. This reflex is helpful during the placement of NG tubes or Ph probes (Wolf and Glass, 1992).

[3] Saint-Anne Dargassies, 1977

The Source for Pediatric Dysphagia

Chapter 2: Medical Disorders, *continued*

Methods of Nutrition

Since premature infants do not have all the skills required for successful feeding and some are so medically fragile they cannot tolerate oral feeding, premature infants are frequently fed via orogastric or nasogastric tubes or may receive nutrition via PEG tubes. All of these are considered *enteral* methods of feeding as the food travels through the gastrointestinal tract. These methods may also be described as *gavage feedings*. Infants whose gastrointestinal systems are impaired may be given nutrition *parenterally* through peripheral or central lines.

Gavage feedings can deprive infants of sucking pleasure and can increase aversive stimulation to the mouth, pharynx, and esophagus, which can lead to oral hypersensitivity. Therefore, it is important to provide pleasurable oral experiences to the infant via non-nutritive sucking (NNS) even if the infant is NPO (nothing by mouth). The sucking reflex diminishes if sucking is not reinforced through nutritive sucking (NS) or NNS experiences (Wolf et al., 1992).

Nutrition in the Pre-term Infant

Pre-term infants have considerably different nutritional requirements than those of a full-term infant. Specifically, protein, calories, calcium, and phosphorous are required in much higher amounts for pre-term babies. Nutritional intake should be monitored by a registered dietician.

Protein	Protein requirements for a pre-term infant are greater than for a full-term infant. Recommendations vary depending on the route of feeding. Term infants require 2.2 grams of protein per kilogram whereas pre-term infants on enteral nutrition require 3.5-4.0 grams of protein per kilogram (AAPCON, 1998). Pre-term infants on parenteral nutrition require slightly less (2.5-3.5 grams of protein per kilogram). Excessive protein intake may be detrimental to the pre-term infant because of renal and metabolic immaturity. Too little protein will impair growth.
Calories	A visual exam of a pre-term infant illustrates low body fat stores. Because of this, and other reasons related to prematurity, energy expenditure in the pre-term infant is greater. Calorie requirements in the pre-term infant are 120 kcals per kilogram vs. 108 kcals per kilogram in the term infant (Groh-Wargo, 1994)
Calcium/ Phosphorous	Premature infants are at risk of osteopenia of prematurity (i.e., decreased bone mass). This impaired bone mineralization can lead to rickets and bone fractures. Risk factors include less than 34 weeks gestation, less than 1500

Chapter 2: Medical Disorders, *continued*

grams birth weight, delayed full feedings enterally, use of term formulas or unfortified breast milk, chronic use of medications that increase mineral excretion, and cholestatic jaundice (Groh-Wargo, 1994).

Pre-term infants often do not accumulate enough calcium and phosphorous, so these nutrients need to be supplemented and appropriate labs and/or radiographs monitored. Enteral nutrition is the most effective means to provide these mineral requirements. Pre-term formulas and breast milk fortifiers are supplemented with calcium and phosphorous and are more appropriate for pre-term infants than term formula or unfortified breast milk.

Nutritive and Non-Nutritive Sucking

Nutritive sucking (NS) occurs at a rate of one suck per second. NS has a longer sucking burst (up to three minutes), uses more negative pressure, and increases jaw depression when compared to non-nutritive sucking (NNS) (Wolff, 1968).

NNS is faster (two sucks per second) and has shorter bursts and pauses. Rhythmic alternation of suction/expression is observed in NNS before it is seen in NS (Lau et al., 1996).

NNS provides many benefits. It can be used after feeding to ease behavior distress reactions. Gill (1988) reported that NNS also increases oxygen levels in the blood, decreases the heart rate, and increases weight gain.

Many experts recommend pairing NNS with gavage feeds. Pickler et al. (1993) reported an increased readiness for bottle feeding and a faster transition when NNS is paired with gavage feeds. DiPietro et al. (found in Lau et al., 1996) compared pre-term infants receiving gavage feedings without accompanying NNS to infants who were provided with NNS opportunities during gavage feedings. When NNS was paired with gavage feeds, it had a soothing effect on the premature infants. The premature infants showed fewer behavioral distress signs and fewer defensive behaviors (e.g., less grimacing, squirming, and thrashing). The premature infants also spent less time in fussy states and returned to stable sleep states faster.

Some infants experience nipple confusion when they transfer from NNS (e.g., pacifier) to NS (e.g., bottles). To reduce possible nipple confusion when transitioning to the bottle, expose the infant to a variety of pacifier shapes. Be sure to include one shaped like the nipple you anticipate using on the bottle (Wolf and Glass, 1992). It is impossible to predict exactly which nipple will be used on the bottle because there are many factors to consider (e.g., size, flow rate).

Chapter 2: Medical Disorders, *continued*

Introducing Oral Feeding

Frequently, premature infants have not achieved a suck-swallow-breathe ratio of 1-1-1 and, therefore, the swallowing pattern is asynchronous. In order to protect the airway, the premature infant attempts to block the nipple with her tongue to stop the flow of milk. Premature infants will also alternate periods of prolonged respiration pauses with periods of sucking during feeding.

Many premature infants have decreased grooving or cupping of the tongue. Tongue grooving or cupping is necessary for an infant to latch on to a nipple.

It is important to try a variety of nipples to determine how the infant does best. A firm nipple will help the infant cup the tongue, latch on to the nipple, and have control of the flow. High flow and soft nipples can increase flow as well as increase aspiration risk due to the infant's inability to coordinate sucking, swallowing, and breathing (Shaker, 1990). If nipple feeding is introduced too early, the premature infant may be exerting too much energy and reducing the calorie intake.

An infant may be ready for oral feeding at 32 weeks, but will be more successful closer to 34 weeks. The pre-term infant also needs to be tolerating gavage feedings, have a stable respiratory status, have a respiratory rate of less than 70, and should not have labored breathing at rest (Wolf and Glass, 1992).

Gastroesophageal Reflux Disease

Gastroesophageal Reflux Disease (GERD) is defined as the contents of the stomach (including stomach acid) being returned to the esophagus. It occurs when the lower esophageal sphincter (LES) does not work properly.

GERD does not only occur during eating and swallowing. It often occurs during transient increases in intra-abdominal pressure above the pressure of the LES, resulting in stomach contents back flowing into the esophagus. These transient increases mainly occur while the child is awake during normal activities like crying, coughing, moving, and defecating.

Individuals with gastrostomy tubes may develop significant GERD after placement of the tube (as many as 12-50%). GERD tends to develop within 6-12 months following tube placement.

Infants and children with GERD may exhibit certain symptoms that might raise suspicion that they have GERD. They may:

- vomit — Many children with GERD have projectile vomiting. (It is not necessary to demonstrate vomiting to have GERD.)

Chapter 2: Medical Disorders, continued

• cough, choke, and/or gag	may occur during or after feeding
• exhibit abnormal posturing	Children with GERD may arch their backs. This may mean they also have esophagitis, or may mean they are distressed because of airway compromise related to the reflux.
• exhibit irritability	Unexplained irritability may be due to GERD.

Infants and children with GERD can develop a variety of clinical manifestations of GERD. These disorders may be caused directly by GERD or may be related to GERD without a specific causal relationship.

Respiratory complications

- recurrent aspiration
- recurrent pneumonia
- chronic cough
- laryngospasm
- laryngitis
- apnea
- reactive airway disease
- bronchopulmonary dysplasia
- stridor
- reflux induced bronchospasm

Esophageal/Gastroenterologic complications

- hematemesis
- anemia
- esophageal spasm
- melena
- strictures
- atresia

Failure to thrive

As mentioned earlier, reflux often occurs during activities like coughing. Therefore, it is not surprising that the following respiratory disorders (accompanied by frequent coughing) can cause reflux or increase frequency of reflux because of an increase in abdominal pressure.

- cystic fibrosis
- bronchopulmonary dysplasia
- asthma

GERD is also more likely if the pressure in the LES is lower than normal. Medications for respiratory disorders and NG tubes can lower pressure in the LES.

The amount of reflux can also be increased if the child is receiving chest physiotherapy or is left in a supine position.

Chapter 2: Medical Disorders, continued

Medical Tests to Diagnose GERD

There are several procedures used to diagnose GERD.

Barium Swallow	Allows physicians to rule out structural problems, but has false positive and false negative rates.
Scintigraphy or Scintiscan	Child ingests radioisotopes and is scanned over the period of an hour. Provides evidence of gastric emptying, esophageal motility, and pulmonary aspiration.
Extended Esophageal pH Monitoring	Most sensitive to determine GERD. Probe remains in place above LES over a period of 24 hours. Quantifies the amount of GERD and helps relate the occurrence of GERD with symptoms (e.g., Does GERD occur when the child shows increased irritability?).
Upper Endoscopy	Allows visualization of the mucosa of the esophagus.

Management of GERD

GERD can be managed behaviorally, medically, or surgically. Speech-language pathologists (SLPs) are generally involved with behavioral management.

Behavioral Management

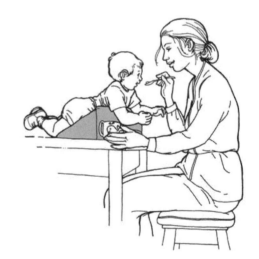

- Position at 30° prone upright on incline. This keeps the contents of the stomach anterior while the LES is superior and posterior.

- Thickened feedings of one teaspoon cereal per ounce seems to reduce the frequency of vomiting.

- Smaller, more frequent feedings throughout the day to keep the stomach from becoming overfull.

- Fasting before bed.

The Source for Pediatric Dysphagia

Chapter 2: Medical Disorders, continued

Medical Management

This is usually not started unless the child does not respond to behavioral management or significant complications of GERD are noted. The three most commonly prescribed types of drugs and the intended effect are:

- bethanechol (Urecholine®) — increases LES pressure and improves esophageal clearance

- metoclopramide (Reglan®) — increases amplitude of peristaltic contractions in the esophagus; elevates resting tone of LES; stimulates gastric emptying

- H2-receptor antagonists include cimetidine (Tagamet®), rantidine (Zantac®), famotidine (Pepcid®) and nizatidine (Axid®) — inhibits nocturnal acid secretion

GERD has also been linked to bronchopulmonary dysplasia and to a chronic cough that sounds like bronchitis or asthma (Herbst, 1981; Orenstein and Orenstein, 1988). Some children cough and choke or exhibit apnea or laryngospasms. GERD has also been linked to respiratory arrest, sudden infant death syndrome (SIDS), and other apparent life-threatening events (ALTEs) (See, 1989). There is often no evidence of gross aspiration in babies with SIDS or apnea. It is hypothesized that laryngospasm or reflux central apnea may be the reason respiratory arrest occurs. It is also possible that stridor is related to gastro-esophageal reflux. It is thought that acid may cause inflammation in the larynx and result in stridor (Nielson et al., 1990).

Surgical Management

Surgical management of GERD in children is not typically needed because GERD usually resolves over time in children up to 18 months of age. If surgery is needed, the procedure often used is Nissen fundoplication. In this surgery, the fundus of the stomach is wrapped around the distal end of the esophagus to provide a tighter sphincter. This is intended to keep the contents of the stomach from flowing back into the esophagus.

Short Bowel Syndrome

Short bowel syndrome is the inability to absorb nutrients and the resulting malnutrition that occurs after a massive resection of the small intestine. In infants, a resection usually has to be done as a result of one of the following disorders:

Chapter 2: Medical Disorders, continued

- multiple intestinal atresias
- intestinal malrotation
- necrotizing enterocolitis
- abdominal wall defects

These children are often maintained on Total Parenteral Nutrition (TPN). TPN provides nutrition via a central line that delivers nutrition to the bloodstream rather than through the gastrointestinal tract.

In order for the remaining intestine to function, the child must begin some oral or enteral feedings. If the child has developed an aversion to food, as is often the case for children receiving only TPN, they may need a PEG tube. These children may be given anti-motility drugs such as loperamide (Imodium®) or diphenoxylate and atropine (Lomotil®) to slow the movement of nutrients through the remaining intestinal tract. This allows more time for the nutrients to be dissolved through the intestinal wall (Rossi, 1993).

Some children with very short intestinal segments can be weaned from TPN after several years, but may continue to need some TPN.

Acquired Immunodeficiency System (AIDS)

Dysphagia is a problem typically found in children with AIDS. In one study (Pressman and Morrison, 1998), more than 45% of pediatric AIDS patients had dysphagia. Seventy-six percent of those patients showed some improvement with treatment.

Pressman (1995) describes two general types of neurological etiologies for the dysphagia associated with AIDS in children.

Static encephalopathy	developmental delay with non-progressive motor deficits, microcephaly, and seizure disorder
Progressive encephalopathy	neurological deterioration due to direct brain infection with HIV

Children might also have a stroke or lesion of the central nervous system as a result of AIDS.

Odynophagia

Odynophagia (i.e., pain with swallowing) may be due to damage of the esophageal mucosa that occurs after repeated infections. Infants may begin to take a bottle and take only one or two sucks on a bottle before stopping and crying if they are experiencing esophageal mucosal damage.

Malnutrition

Children with AIDS may experience malnutrition which in turn affects many other systems in the body and may place the child at risk for aspiration. It may also result in increased fatigue during eating.

Children may present as very slow feeders with poor sucking, chewing, and bolus formation. These children may also develop an aversion to food because textured foods were not introduced early enough.

Phases Affected

Since neurological disorders can cause different types of dysphagia, oral preparatory, oral voluntary, and pharyngeal phases of the swallow may all be affected in children with AIDS. Esophageal phase disorders (e.g., mucosal injury) may also occur.

Effects of AIDS Drugs

The drugs used to treat AIDS and the complications of AIDS may cause other dysphagia symptoms. Some side effects of the medications include:
- nausea
- vomiting
- increased reflux (resulting in decreased acceptance of foods)
- decreased appetite

Some Tips on Treatment

Pressman (1995) provides the following tips concerning the treatment of children with dysphagia. These may be helpful in addition to other oral-motor treatment or dietary changes described in Chapter 5.

Children with chronic pain

Give a mild analgesic about 20 minutes prior to a meal. This may improve the amount and type of food the child will accept.

Children with cardiac or respiratory problems who take oxygen

Increase the flow of oxygen during feedings.

Children refusing medications secondary to taste

Put the medicine in a spoonful of pudding or other flavorful food.

Chapter 2: Medical Disorders, continued

Children with odynophagia

Use smooth, cold foods (e.g., pudding, ice cream). Avoid strong flavored or acidic foods (e.g., tomatoes, oranges) or foods with sharp edges (e.g., hard cookies, potato chips).

Cerebral Palsy

Cerebral Palsy (CP) is the most common cause of congenital neurogenic dysphagia (Christiansen, 1989). CP is a movement and/or posture disorder that is the result of an encepalopathy that occurs prenatally, perinatally, or during childhood. Many children with CP maintain primitive and/or abnormal reflexes. Children with CP often grow poorly, even to the point of being diagnosed with failure to thrive.

Types of Swallowing Problems

Children with CP may have increased tone (hypertonic), decreased tone (hypotonic), or fluctuating tone as in athetosis. Most children with CP will have dysphagia related to poor lip and tongue function which may result in a weak suck, inability to drink effectively from a cup, and decreased ability to chew and form a bolus and to manipulate the bolus in the mouth. These children may also have a delayed swallow which puts them at risk for aspiration. Increased pharyngeal residue also places them at risk for aspiration.

Other problems which interfere with the oral phase of dysphagia include tongue thrust, tonic bite reflex, strong gag, and hypersensitivity in the mouth and face. Children with CP maintain suckle and rooting responses beyond the age of six months.

GERD

GERD is thought to occur in up to 75% of children with CP. This may occur because of abnormal peristalsis and impaired function of the LES. Many children with CP may experience lung disease caused by reflux, as well as colic esophagitis with painful swallowing, anemia, and formation of strictures.

Behavioral Feeding Disorders

Children with severe CP may acquire a behavioral feeding disorder (Chapter 8) as a result of repeated unpleasant experiences associated with feeding (e.g., vomiting, choking, having NG tubes inserted). These negative experiences cause the child to learn to refuse to take anything orally or perhaps to develop an aversion to stimulation around the mouth. This may lead to the need for placement of a feeding tube. One study found that rapid improvement of nutritional

Chapter 2: Medical Disorders, continued

intake via NG or gastrostomy tube led to improvement in circulation, healing, mood, and spasticity (Patrick et al., 1986).

Pulmonary Function

Christiansen (1989) points out that respiratory infections are one of the most common causes of death for children with severe neuro-developmental handicaps (e.g., CP, microcephaly). Children with CP are at risk for aspiration because of poor coordination of swallowing and breathing. In addition, the fact that many of these children are immobile, have weak muscles of respiration, and a poor protective cough means that they are more susceptible to developing pneumonia and other respiratory disorders as a result of aspiration.

Aspiration

A child with CP who has aspirated may cough or show distress, or may have recurrent wheezing or rattly breathing. Aspiration in an infant can cause apnea. Older children with CP who have experienced aspiration over a period of months or years may have severe lung problems such as interstitial fibrosis, bronchiolitis, and persistent atelectasis (Phelan et al., 1990). Children may also be silent aspirators, similar to adults.

Treatment Effects

Several studies in the literature document the effectiveness of initiating treatment with children with CP, even when the children present with profound retardation and severe CP. Some examples of those findings are reported here.

Helfrich-Miller et al. (1986) describe six patients with profound CP, ages 12-31, who were examined through videofluoroscopy. Programs consisting of dietary modifications, oral-motor treatment, and thermal stimulation were initiated. Results showed significant gain in pharyngeal transit time, amount of material aspirated, amount of residue in valleculae and pyriform sinuses, and the number of swallows required to clear the oropharynx. The patients were capable of making gains in swallowing function based upon what is described as a passive treatment paradigm.

Ammundson et al. (1994) highlight the importance of a complete assessment by a registered dietician and stress the importance of frequent monitoring to prevent malnutrition. They state that malnutrition associated with poor oral intake, gastroesophageal reflux with aspiration, and chronic constipation were frequent management issues in individuals with severe disabilities.

Gisel et al. (1994, '95, '96) describe the effects of treatment with children with CP. An examination of 35 children, ages four to 13 years, found that after 20 weeks of sensory motor treatment, limited improvement was observed in spoon

Chapter 2: Medical Disorders, continued

feeding, biting, and chewing, but not in drinking. The children maintained their pre-treatment weight/age percentile. The authors concluded that to meet the increasing demands of the teenage years, oral-motor therapy may need to be combined with oral-caloric supplementation.

The 1996 study by Gisel et al. again found some improvement in spoon feeding, chewing, and swallowing, but no significant change in drinking skills. They also found that children who received treatment seemed to ingest food more completely (e.g., less spillage), but their weight remained at the lowest age norms.

Children with spastic quadriplegia have the highest rates of associated deficits, including mental retardation and memory deficits. Their oral-motor dysfunction mirrors the degree of dysfunction in the extremities. Significant dysphagia is commonly observed in children with quadriplegia or extrapyramidal forms of CP (Capute et al., 1991).

Head Injury

Patients with head injury with dysphagia require stays in rehabilitation hospitals twice as long as those without dysphagia (Field and Weiss, 1989).

Nutritional Needs During Coma

Nutritional needs significantly increase during the period of coma. The Basal Metabolic Rate (BMR) is influenced by coma status. For instance, Clifton et al. (1986) point out that patients with decorticate/decerebrate posturing indicating a deep coma show 20% higher basal energy expenditures than patients who are localizing painful stimuli, which suggests that they are beginning to recover from the coma.

Following severe head trauma, children enter a phase described as highly catabolic with an increase in their resting metabolic rate of 130-140% above what you would expect in an individual of the same age, weight, and size who is not injured. During this phase, the patient must be given calories at 1½ times the predicted rate of energy expenditure to prevent breakdown of body tissue and to promote rebuilding (Epstein et al., 1987). It is beyond the scope of this book to discuss the many other complex factors concerning maintaining adequate nutrition and hydration during comas.

Comparison of Dysphagia in Children and Adults

Children with head injuries appear to have dysphagic symptoms that are very similar to adults who have experienced head injuries. Their dysphagia often includes poor ability to manipulate a bolus related to decreased tongue control and delayed pharyngeal swallow.

Chapter 2: Medical Disorders, *continued*

Yvilsaker and Weinstein (1989) point out a number of differences between children and adults that can affect the recovery of oral feeding after a head injury.

- The differences in anatomy and physiology between infants, older children, and adults as explained in Chapter 1.

- The different requirements for nutrition and hydration for children and adults.

- The likelihood that significant cognitive/behavioral issues will interfere with re-establishing oral feeding in children.

- The social impact on the family in feeding a child with dysphagia poses a significant challenge.

Yvilsaker and Weinstein indicate that changes in anatomy and physiology, differing requirements for nutrition and hydration, and cognitive behavioral issues interfere more with recovery of swallowing in children than adults. Many of the treatment techniques described in Chapter 5 apply, but it is important to determine if the child with a cognitive deficit related to a head injury is going to be able to follow the directions for safe eating. The child must be able to follow simple commands, probably at least at a Rancho Level III.[1] Children who have experienced head injury may be very impulsive, taking large bites and failing to chew and swallow before taking another bite. In addition, when children are in a confused or agitated state, they may refuse food.

Videofluoroscopic Evaluation

Yvilsaker and Weinstein caution that the timing of videofluoroscopic evaluation of swallowing in a child recovering from a head injury is quite sensitive. If the child is in a phase with increased oral hypersensitivity and aggression, it may not be the best time to complete the evaluation. As would be recommended when evaluating any child using videofluoroscopy, it is important to help the child with a head injury become comfortable in the situation. Explain what is going to happen and let the child look at, touch, and feel comfortable with the equipment before the study begins. Have the child's parent(s) with her during the study if at all possible.

GERD

Arvedson (1993) indicates that GERD is fairly common in children with head injuries and may be even more evident after placement of an NG tube.

---

[1] Hagen, C., Malkmus, D., and Durham, P., *Levels of Cognitive Functioning*. Rancho Los Amigos Medical Center, Downey, CA, 1971

Chapter 2: Medical Disorders, continued

Treatment Suggestions

In addition to the treatment techniques found in Chapter 5, Arvedson (1993) suggests other things to keep in mind about children who have experienced head injuries:

- Upright positioning may not always be possible. Yvilsaker and Weinstein (1989) suggest a position which is semi-reclined, but maintains the 90° angle of trunk and limbs and a slight chin tuck.

- Tube feeding should be continued until it is clear that the child is going to be able to take enough food by mouth.

- Proceed very cautiously, especially with children in the early stages of coma recovery because they are easily agitated.

- It may be necessary to reduce oral hypersensitivity. Begin tactile stimulation on the trunk or limbs and gradually move toward the hypersensitive oral area.

- Early coma stimulation techniques such as improving awareness and alertness and increasing appropriate response to sensory stimulation will provide a basis for more specific feeding treatment at a later time.

- A child with an absent swallow reflex presents a particular challenge, as she often will not let you work in the oral cavity with a laryngeal mirror. A technique such as neurosensory stimulation may be more easily administered. This involves filling the finger of a glove with water, tying it off, and freezing it. You can also fill the finger with crushed ice. The child can then suck on it to elicit a pharyngeal swallow. This way, the child gets the cold stimulation and the sucking motion without being given anything by mouth.

- If the child has a bite reflex, use a rubber-coated spoon or even a NUK® rubber infant toothbrush to present the initial tastes of food.

- Consider the environment in which feeding therapy occurs. It should be quiet and free of distraction.

Goal of Treatment

The desired goal of treatment, of course, is to return the child to full PO intake. However, that may not be possible with some children because of their degree of impairment. In that case, other goals as highlighted by Yvilsaker and Logemann (1985) include:

1. oral feeding with compensatory techniques or a restricted range of food types and textures

Chapter 2: Medical Disorders, continued

2. a combination of oral and tube feeding with the tube used primarily to maintain hydration

3. minimal "recreational" feeding for long-term severely-involved patients

Fetal Alcohol Syndrome

Children with Fetal Alcohol Syndrome present with multiple physical problems and craniofacial disorders. They may also have microcephaly, mental retardation, or other abnormalities. These children may need NG feeding because of poor suck, fatigue, and distractibility. Arvedson (1993) indicated that children may not reach complete oral feeding until after one year of age.

Airway Feeding Problems

Choanal Stenosis-Atresia

Bilateral Choanal Stenosis-Atresia affects one in 5,000 newborns (Brodsky and Volk, 1994). This disorder, in which gross nasal passages are closed, may show up at the first attempt at feeding. Since children breathe through their noses when they are swallowing for approximately the first six months of their life, the child becomes cyanotic when she tries to feed. This does not resolve until the child begins to cry, opens her mouth, and breathes through her mouth. Cothoanal Stenosis-Atresia is usually treated with surgical repair to provide an open nasal airway.

CHARGE Association

Some children have Choanal Stenosis-Atresia as a part of a multiple congenital anomaly known as CHARGE association. The acronym *CHARGE* was coined in 1982 by Pagon et al., and refers to a complex of malformations that include:

Coloboma
Heart disease
Atresia Choanae
Retarded growth and/or development
Genital hypoplasia
Ear anomalies and/or deafness

This array of symptoms is thought to be secondary to the abnormal development of the neural crest during embryogenesis (Asher et al., 1990). Because these babies have developmental delays, it is not surprising to note that many have feeding disorders as well.

Chapter 2: Medical Disorders, continued

Pierre Robin (also see Craniofacial Anomalies, pages 50-53)

Children with Pierre Robin have a mandibular hypoplasia, glossoptosis (tongue falling back into the airway), and cleft palate. These children may not exhibit airway obstruction until they begin feeding. Shprintzen (1988) indicates there are three reasons for airway obstruction in mandibular hypoplasia:

- glossoptosis during inspiration

- palatal shelves drawn inward which obstruct the airway

- lateral pharyngeal wall hypotonia causes pharyngeal or hypopharyngeal collapse

These problems may be treated by surgically affixing the tongue to the lip (a procedure called *glossopexy*), use of nasopharyngeal tubes to maintain an airway, or tracheotomy.

Tracheo-Esophageal Fistulae/Esophageal Atresia

Tracheo-Esophageal Fistula (TEF) are openings which occur between the esophagus and the trachea. This is a common congenital anomaly with the incidence varying between one in 1,500 to one in 4,500 live births (Anderson et al., 1979). These infants previously had a near 100% mortality. At present, they exhibit a survival rate of 80%, with survival reaching 100% in infants who weigh 2700 grams or more at birth (Rosen et al., 1984).

TEF and Esophageal Atresia (EA) are classified as different types, depending on where the esophagus ends and where and how the fistula with the trachea occurs.

Type A
EA without fistula. The proximal end of the esophagus does not attach to the distal end. There are two blind pouches and neither connects to the trachea.

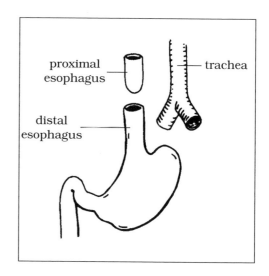

Chapter 2: Medical Disorders, *continued*

Type B
TEF to the proximal end of the esophagus. The top of the esophagus connects to the trachea.

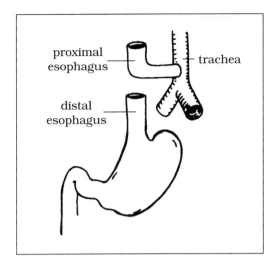

Type C
EA with fistula to the distal end of the esophagus. The top of the esophagus ends in a blind pouch, but the distal end of the esophagus attaches to the trachea.

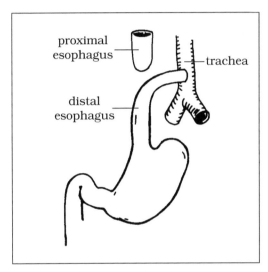

Type D
EA with fistula to both ends of the esophagus. The proximal and distal ends of the esophagus attach to the trachea.

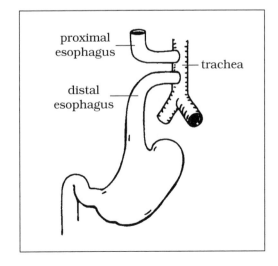

Chapter 2: Medical Disorders, continued

Type E (also called **Type H**)
TEF without atresia. The distal and proximal ends of the esophagus are attached to one another, but there is also an opening into the trachea. The opening can be very small. This type of TEF is often not discovered right away as the infant is able to eat, but food/liquid enters the airway.

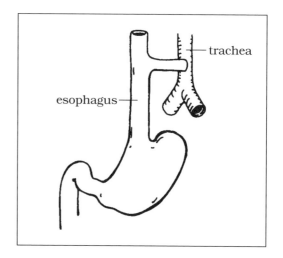

There are several options for surgical repair of TEF/EA. With most types of TEF/EA, infants cannot eat until surgical repair occurs. After surgery, these infants may develop some esophageal stenosis at the site. They may require repeated esophageal dilatations.

Infants with this problem may have long-term complications according to the type of defect, type of surgical repair, and structural characteristics. Some of the problems they may encounter include:

- tracheomalacia — an abnormality of the trachea that causes it to be unstable and prone to collapse

- esophageal dismotility — food and liquid move too slowly through the esophagus after repair, making the child at risk for aspiration

- formation of strictures — some degree of narrowing at the site where the two sections of the esophagus are joined

- GERD — with increased risk of aspiration and decreased intake of food

- respiratory complications — related to aspiration

- nutritional deficits — cannot take in enough food

SLPs may see these infants before surgical repair to assure that oral-motor skills are developed through non-nutritive sucking and to decrease hypersensitivity of the face and mouth. Hypersensitivity may develop because these infants are subjected to placement of tubes for feeding and are suctioned frequently. After surgical repair, the infant can begin eating and SLPs may begin feeding therapy.

Chapter 2: Medical Disorders, continued

Laryngeal Anomalies

Children may present with a number of laryngeal anomalies that can lead to feeding difficulties. These may include vocal cord paralysis, supraglottic growth, abnormalities of the epiglottis, subglottic stenosis, and laryngeal cleft. Most of these require surgical intervention.

Bronchopulmonary Dysplasia

Bronchopulmonary dysplasia (BPD) is the leading cause of infant lung disease in the United States and affects approximately 7,000 newborn infants annually (Northway, 1990). Infants with BPD have biological risk factors that may interfere with the acquisition of normal feeding behaviors and may negatively effect long-term growth and development. They have an elevated resting metabolic rate and rapid respiratory rate with episodes of hypoxemia, especially while sleeping. This may result in poor oxygenation for metabolic needs. These infants may respond to increased oxygen supplementation.

Infants with BPD may also have neurologic abnormalities, difficulties coordinating sucking and swallowing, and an increased incidence of GERD. All of these things may interfere with the child receiving adequate nutrition. These infants are also intolerant of fluids. They often become overloaded on fluids and require diuretic therapy. Diuretic therapy has many complications, such as diarrhea or causing infant respiratory distress. BPD is sometimes treated by restricting fluids or using high carbohydrate loads in formulas.

Feeding problems are common in infants with BPD and stem from ongoing respiratory problems as well as behaviorally-based problems resulting from significant number of medical intervention procedures. Wolf and Glass (1992) point out that the most important factor in children with BPD is achieving adequate nutrition. Sometimes oral feeding only leads to marginal nutrition and causes the child to expend too much energy. If that is the case, the child should be maintained without any oral feeding. These infants often have significantly reduced endurance and may also have poor coordination of sucking, swallowing, and breathing. These infants may also exhibit abnormal oral-motor patterns with wide jaw excursion and poorly coordinated tongue movements with a bunched or humped tongue.

Infants with BPD may also struggle to breathe adequately whether on or off the ventilator and may adopt a strong neck extension position. This may be what causes the wide jaw excursion and tongue protrusion.

These infants also have lengthy intubations for mechanical ventilation and may suffer some laryngeal injury. Paschley and Fan (1988) report moderate to major injury to the larynx in 44-55% of infants who were intubated. If laryngeal dysfunction with pharyngeal phase dysphagia is suspected, these infants may need videofluoroscopic evaluation of swallowing.

Chapter 2: Medical Disorders, *continued*

Tracheostomy

Infants with BPD, subglottic stenosis, or tracheomalcia may require a tracheostomy. If it is anticipated that the child will need long-term ventilation, a tracheostomy is preferred to oral intubation. Some children need a tracheostomy, but may not require assisted ventilation.

A tracheostomy does not have any effect on oral skills, but it is often placed after the infant has had long-term oral intubation. In that case, the child may already have developed hypersensitivity of the face and oral cavity. If the child has had prolonged oral intubation, she will not have had an opportunity to practice oral skills through sucking.

Presence of the tracheostomy tube can limit laryngeal elevation which is necessary for achieving airway closure. In addition, the tracheostomy tube prevents air from traveling through the larynx and the larynx may become desensitized. Infants who are mechanically ventilated may not have learned how to coordinate sucking, swallowing, and breathing since the ventilator may control the timing of breathing. When they are weaned from the ventilator, they may need to learn these skills. Even if the child is not ready to take oral feedings, it is important that the child experience some pleasurable oral interaction such as non-nutritive sucking and oral stimulation. This may help prevent the child from becoming totally aversive to facial and oral stimulation.

Congenital Heart Disease

There are many classifications of congenital heart disease. The incidence is eight per 1,000 live births (Park, 1984). In 50% of the occurrences, congenital heart disease is an isolated defect. In other cases, it occurs with other problems such as chromosomal defects and syndromes. Wolf and Glass (1992) classify cardiovascular defects as:

- abnormal connections between the systemic and pulmonary vascular systems

- obstruction of the normal blood flow through the heart

- a combination of the two

Infants with congenital heart disease may show significantly decreased endurance. Because of this, they will not eat enough and seem to lack a hunger drive. They often do not wake up spontaneously for their feedings and seem uninterested in eating. They may respond with aversive behaviors such as gagging if pushed to eat. Techniques which may be helpful for these infants include:

- providing chin or cheek support to help increase the strength of the suck

- using a nipple which allows more fluid to flow

Chapter 2: Medical Disorders, *continued*

- giving frequent breaks

- consulting with a dietitian about formula that has higher density of calories and nutrients

Failure to Thrive

Failure to thrive (FTT) is a term used to describe children whose weight is consistently below the third percentile for age, or is less than 80% of the ideal weight for age (Arvedson, 1993). FTT can be classified into organic, non-organic, or mixed etiology.

Some of the organic causes include endocrine deficiencies, chronic disease, enzymatic defects, or congenital or genetic anomalies. In addition, oral-motor dysfunction may be another organic cause of FTT. Children who are difficult to feed often do not get adequate nutrition.

Contributing factors in non-organic FTT include poor mother-infant interaction, psycho-social issues, environmental deprivation, child abuse, and poor feeding practices. Many children who have been diagnosed as FTT have developmental disabilities as well. Sometimes FTT and resultant inadequate nutrition cause the developmental disability. Other times, the developmental disability may be the reason the child cannot get adequate nutrition. Non-organic FTT is often associated with a disturbed mother-child relationship. Lachenmeyer (1995) lists maternal factors that have been associated with non-organic FTT:

- lack of nutritional information
- improper feeding techniques
- unrealistic expectations about feeding
- inability to accurately assess the child's needs
- neglect
- isolation

Lachenmeyer (1995) indicates that assessment should include asking the caregiver to keep a daily food intake diary. (See Chapter 8, page 205.) She suggests it should include the time the food was eaten, behaviors associated with intake, and the quantity eaten. Lachenmeyer describes this as baseline information against which to measure progress. She also asks the family to record routines. With this diary, a determination can be made whether attempts to feed throughout the day are disrupting other aspects of family life.

More information about specific approaches to use with infants with FTT are found in Chapter 8 on behavioral aspects of feeding disorders.

Chapter 2: Medical Disorders, continued

Craniofacial Anomalies

Feeding difficulties may occur in infants with cleft palate and/or cleft lip and in infants with other craniofacial anomalies. These difficulties are apparent from birth when the infant tries to nurse or suck a bottle. It is important that these children receive immediate intervention to prevent deficits in nutrition.

Cleft Palate

A cleft palate prevents a child from creating negative pressure while sucking. The inability to seal off the nasal cavity from the oral cavity is the main cause of this inability to suck adequately. Typically, these infants have a normal sucking movement and rhythm, but they can't build up negative intraoral pressure. This results in excessive amounts of air during nipple feeding which causes the infant to become uncomfortable from bloating. They may also experience choking and gagging as well as fatigue because it takes them so long to complete a feeding. Any and all of these may contribute to lack of weight gain.

Cleft Lip

Children with cleft lip experience difficulty achieving lip seal against the nipple, but this is a relatively minor problem compared to the cleft palate. Children with cleft lip only are often able to feed adequately.

Submucous Cleft

A submucous cleft may be related to velopharyngeal insufficiency. If so, the child may have nasopharyngeal reflux.

Surgical Repair

Clefts of the lip are typically repaired surgically between one and three months of age (Weatherly-White, 1990). Most surgeons wait to perform the surgery until the child weighs about ten pounds. Primary repair of the cleft of the palate is typically done between six and 12 months of age. These surgical procedures have temporary negative effects on the child's feeding ability.

Feeding Tips and Techniques

Arvedson (1993) summarizes basic changes which can be made in feeding to help improve the efficiency and effectiveness in feeding infants with cleft palate.

Positioning

Children with cleft palate typically respond better when fed in an upright position with support given to the trunk, neck, and head. This keeps the liquid from running too quickly into the posterior oral cavity which can cause choking. It also reduces entry of formula into the nasal cavity and eustachian tubes during sucking.

Nipple

A nipple with a soft, thin wall that the child can easily compress is most helpful. Cross-cut nipples allow fluid to flow more easily with less pressure. Some infants respond better to a wide, flat nipple such as a NUK®. There is a balance between making sure that enough liquid flows in so the infant can compensate for her weak suck, and keeping the flow slow enough that the infant doesn't choke.

In the past, nurses and physicians recommended a lamb's nipple. This seems to be contraindicated in infants with cleft palate. A lamb's nipple is too long and it releases the fluid too posteriorly in the oral cavity. Nipples with a wide base allow children with cleft lip to seal onto the nipple better. The wide base of the nipple accommodates for the opening in the lip.

Burping

Infants with cleft palates need frequent burping.

Frequency of Feeding

Feeding will take longer than with the typical infant. These infants may take 20-30 minutes to feed and will probably need to be fed at two- to four-hour intervals.

Type of Bottle

The Haberman Feeder® is designed specifically for infants with cleft palate. It has a one-way valve that allows easy flow of liquids and prevents backflow. No vacuum is produced, which means it is much easier to suck. The nipple also has three different rates of flow (Haberman, 1988).

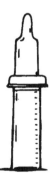

Mead-Johnson also produces a cleft palate nurser. It is a soft bottle, which allows the feeder to squeeze slightly to help the infant get more liquid.

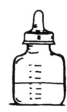

A nurser with a rigid plastic shell and disposable inner plastic bags can also be used. Paradise (1990) describes an adaption of this making two slots in the rigid shell so that a finger can be inserted to squeeze the bag. This then acts in the same way as the Mead-Johnson flexible bottle.

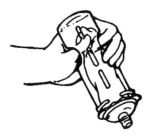

An angle-necked bottle may also be helpful, although none of the bottles described above come in an angled format.

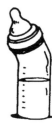

Monitoring Intake

It is important to monitor how much formula the infant is able to take. Infants who are taking only two to three ounces an hour are probably not going to do well in terms of weight gain.

Spoon Feeding

Spoon feeding should be introduced at the same age it would be with a typical child. The baby foods may need to be thinned a bit, as stickier foods tend to cling in the cleft area.

The area around the cleft should be cleaned thoroughly after feeding so food does not accumulate and possibly cause an infection. The area can be cleaned with plain or sterile water on a washcloth or piece of gauze.

Chapter 2: Medical Disorders, *continued*

Breast-feeding in Children with Cleft Lip and Palate

If the child has only a cleft of the lip, she may be able to successfully breast-feed. Some lateral cheek support may be needed to help achieve increased lip closure around the nipple. A small amount of milk leaking anteriorly is not abnormal.

Infants with cleft palate, even if they do not have a cleft lip, have more difficulty breast-feeding. Some infants with clefts of the soft palate may be able to learn to take milk from the breast if the mother provides finger pressure to the breast at the top and bottom edges to make it easier for the infant to take the nipple into her mouth (Grady, 1977). The mother may also need to hold the nipple in the infant's mouth throughout the feeding.

Babies with clefts of the hard palate may not be successful with breast-feeding. Consideration needs to be given to the infant's growth rate, the time required for feeding, and the stress on the infant and the mother in trying this approach.

Wolf and Glass (1992) point out that the anti-bacterial properties of breast milk may be very important for infants with craniofacial anomalies because they experience an increased incidence of otitis media. Even if the infant is unable to drink from the breast, expressed breast milk may be more beneficial than formula.

When working with infants with craniofacial anomalies whose mothers wish to breast-feed, it is important to remember that the flow of milk is different from that which occurs during bottle feeding. In breast-feeding, it can take two minutes of active sucking to elicit the "let-down" reflex which yields strong milk flow. The physical characteristics of the mother's breast must also be considered since there is a wide variation in the size and shape. The infant has to be able to latch on well for successful breast-feeding to occur.

Feeding After Surgery

In the first 24 hours after surgery, feeding is by cup or syringe so the child does not have to use a strong suction action. Check with the surgeon for specific recommendations as to when feeding can be resumed. If cup drinking is recommended (even in a younger infant) after lip repair, the infant may have better luck with slightly thickened liquids.

Pierre Robin and Micrognathia
(Also see Airway Feeding Problems, page 43.)

The term *Pierre Robin Syndrome* applies to newborn micrognathia. Three findings are typically included in this description:

- micrognathia

Chapter 2: Medical Disorders, continued

- upper airway obstruction (presumably caused by glossoptosis)
- wide U-shaped cleft palate

However, not all agree that it is necessary to have a cleft palate to be described as having Pierre Robin Syndrome.

Infant mortality in Pierre Robin Syndrome remains high (Dykes et al., 1985). Although there is disagreement on what constitutes all the components of Pierre Robin, it is agreed that micrognathia must exist. It is thought that the abnormally small or abnormally positioned mandible in utero triggers the development of other anomalies. Because the mandible is retracted, the tongue stays pushed back in the mouth and rests against the cranial base which then interferes with the palatal shelves as they try to grow together. This results in a cleft palate.

After birth, the infant keeps her mouth closed and the tongue falls into the pharyngeal airway causing airway obstruction. There is much discussion over what causes the mandible to be small. One hypothesis is that the mandible is small because of not enough space in the uterus which causes the fetus to flex with her head to her chest, physically preventing the mandible from growing (Shprintzen, 1988). Sherer et al. (1995) hypothesize that normal mandibular growth may depend on the presence of mandibular movement which occurs during swallowing. They examined 14 fetuses with absent mandibular movement and all had micrognathia.

The term *Pierre Robin* is used loosely to characterize children with one or more of the characteristics listed above. However, all children do not have all symptoms.

Shprintzen (1988) indicates that the term *Pierre Robin* probably should not be used as children who have been grouped together under that diagnostic category are quite heterogeneous. Instead, the child should be described by the symptoms presented.

Effects on Feeding

Because of the micrognathia, the tongue is retracted and is not used effectively to compress a nipple. Until the child has some surgical intervention, the major issue with feeding is in trying to maintain an open airway. When fed in the supine position, as is typical with infants, gravity pulls the tongue into the pharynx and compromises the airway. An open and stable airway has to be established before oral feeding can be considered.

An appropriate nipple for feeding a child with Pierre Robin/micrognathia is one that is long enough to produce contact between the nipple and the tongue so sucking movements are effective. However, the nipple should not be long enough to induce gagging. In order for the nipple to be long enough, you may need to insert it fully (i.e., all the way to the hard plastic ring which affixes the nipple to the bottle) into the infant's mouth. For that reason, a nipple with a narrow base is suggested.

The effectiveness of breast-feeding with micrognathia depends on how impaired the child is and whether an adequate airway can be maintained. It is often difficult for an infant with a recessed jaw to adequately latch on to the nipple.

Upper Airway Obstruction

These infants are usually maintained with NG tube feedings until they have gained sufficient weight to undergo surgery. Glossopexy is a procedure in which the tongue is anchored to the mandible and lower lip. This keeps the tongue out of the oral-pharyngeal airway. Any cleft palate is repaired. These infants also often require tracheostomy.

Another intervention is the use of a naso-pharyngeal (NP) airway tube. This tube is placed behind the tongue and above the epiglottis. Oral feeding can occur when the NP airway is in place, but it is important to maintain appropriate positioning. If the infant is showing distress, or formula is regularly coming through the tube, then the tube is not positioned correctly and should be re-evaluated.

Moëbius Sequence

This sequence of events is characterized by damage to cranial nerves which results in weakness in the lower face, usually affecting the mandible, lips, and tongue. The child has difficulty closing her lips because of the weakness, and food and liquid dribble out of her mouth.

Chapter 2: Medical Disorders, continued

References

AIDS

Pressman, H. "Dysphagia in children with AIDS." In Rosenthal, S. et al. (eds.) *Dysphagia and the Child with Developmental Disabilities: Medical, Clinical, and Family Intervention*, San Diego: Singular Publishing Group, Inc., 1995, p. 135.

Pressman, H. and Morrison, S.H. "Dysphagia in the Pediatric AIDS Population." *Dysphagia*, Vol. 2, 1988, pp. 162-169.

Bronchopulmonary Dysplasia

Kurzener, S.I. et al. "Growth Failure in Infants with Broncopulmonary Dysplasia: Nutrition and Elevated Resting Metabolic Expenditure." *Pediatrics*, Vol. 81, 1988, pp. 379-384.

Northway, W. "Bronchopulmonary Dysplasia: Then and Now." *Archives of Disease in Children*, Vol. 65, 1990, pp. 1076-1081.

Paschley, N.R.T. and Fan, L.L. "Laryngeal Injury from Endo-tracheal Intubation in the Neonate." In Bancalari, E. and Stocker J. T. (eds.) *Bronchopulmonary Dysplasia*, Washington, D.C.: Hemisphere Publishing Corporation, 1988, pp. 211-219.

Pearlman, J.M. and Vole, J.J. "Movement Disorder of Premature Infants with Severe Bronchopulmonary Dysplasia: A New Syndrome." *Pediatrics*, Vol. 84, 1989, pp. 215-218.

Cerebral Palsy

Ammundson, J.A. et al. "Early Identification and Treatment Necessary to Prevent Malnutrition in Children and Adolescents with Severe Disabilities." *Journal of the American Dietetic Association*, Vol. 94, No. 8, 1994, pp. 880-883.

Arvedson, J.C. "Dysphagia in Pediatric Patients with Neurologic Damage." *Seminars in Neurology*, Vol. 16, No. 4, 1996, pp. 371-386.

Capute, A.J. and Acardo, P.G. (eds.) "Cerebral Palsy: The Spectrum of Motor Dysfunction." *Developmental Disabilities in Infants and Childhood*, Baltimore: Paul H. Brookes, 1991, pp. 335-348.

Gisel, E.G. "Oral-Motor Skills Following Sensorimotor Intervention on the Moderately-Impaired with Cerebral Palsy." *Dysphagia*, Vol. 9, 1994, pp. 180-192.

Gisel, E.G. et al. "Effect of Oral Sensorimotor Treatment on Measures of Growth, Eating Efficiency and Aspiration in the Dysphagia Child with Cerebral Palsy." *Developmental Medicine and Child Neurology*, Vol. 37, 1995, pp. 528-543.

Gisel, E.G. et al. "Oral-Motor Skills Following Sensorimotor Therapy in Two Groups of Moderately Dysphagic Children with Cerebral Palsy: Aspiration vs. Non-Aspiration." *Dysphagia*, Vol. 11, 1996, pp. 59-71.

Chapter 2: Medical Disorders, continued

Helfrich-Miller, K.R. et al. "Dysphagia: Its Treatment in the Profoundly Retarded Patient with Cerebral Palsy." *Archives of Physical Medicine and Rehabilitation*, Vol. 67, 1986, pp. 520-525.

Patrick, J. et al. "Rapid Correction of Wasting in Children with Cerebral Palsy." *Developmental Medicine and Child Neurology*, Vol. 28, 1986, pp. 734-739.

CHARGE

Asher, S.A. et al. "Airway Complications in CHARGE Association." *Archives of Otolaryngology Head and Neck Surgery*, Vol. 116, 1990, pp. 594-595.

Brodsky, L. and Volk, M. "The Airway and Swallowing." In Arvedson, J. and Brodsky, L. (eds.) *Pediatric Swallowing and Feeding: Assessment and Management*, San Diego: Singular Publishing Group, Inc., 1993, p. 104.

Congenital Heart Disease

Park, M.K. *Pediatric Cardiology for Practitioners*, Chicago: Yearbook Medical Publishers, 1984.

Craniofacial Anomalies

Anderson, G.C. and Vidyasarga, D. "Development of Sucking in Premature Infants from 1 to 7 Days Post Birth." *Birth Defects: Original Article Series*, Vol. 15, 1979, pp. 145-171.

Arvedson, J. "Feeding with Craniofacial Anomalies." In Arvedson, J. and Brodsky, L. (eds.) *Pediatric Swallowing and Feeding: Assessment and Management*, San Diego: Singular Publishing Group, Inc., 1993, pp. 417-429.

Grady, E. "Breast-feeding the Baby with the Cleft of the Soft Palate." *Clinical Pediatrics*, Vol. 16, 1977, pp. 978-981.

Haberman, M. "A Mother of Invention." *Nursing Times*, Vol. 84, No. 2, 1988, pp. 52-53.

Paradise, J.L. "Primary Care of Infants and Children with Cleft Palate." In Bluestone, C. D. et al. (eds.) *Pediatric Otolaryngology*, 2nd ed. Philadelphia: W. B. Saunders, 1990, pp. 860-866.

Rosen, C.L. et al. "Hypoxemia Associated with Feeding in the Pre-Term Infant and Full-term Neonate." *American Journal of Diseases of Childhood*, Vol. 138, 1984, pp. 623-628.

Weatherly-White, R.C. "Surgical Timing and Post-operative Feeding in the Cleft Lip Child." In Kernahan, D. A. and Rosenstein, F. W. (eds.) *Cleft Lip and Palate: A System of Management*, Baltimore: Williams and Wilkins, 1990, pp. 33-36.

Failure to Thrive

Arvedson, J. "Management of Swallowing Problems." In Arvedson, J. and Brodsky, L. (eds.) *Pediatric Swallowing and Feeding: Assessment and Management*, San Diego: Singular Publishing Group, Inc., 1993, pp. 370-371.

Lachenmeyer, J.R. "Behavior Aspects of Feeding Disorders." In Rosenthal, S. et al. (eds.) *Dysphagia and the Child with Developmental Disabilities: Medical, Clinical and Family Interventions*, San Diego: Singular Publishing Group, Inc., 1995, pp. 143-152.

Chapter 2: Medical Disorders, *continued*

General

Arvedson, J. and Brodsky, L. *Pediatric Swallowing and Feeding: Assessment and Management*, San Diego: Singular Publishing Group, Inc., 1993.

Christiansen, J.R. "Developmental Approach to Pediatric Neurogenic Dysphagia." *Dysphagia*, Vol. 3, 1989, pp. 131-134.

Couriel, J.M. et al. "Assessment of Feeding Problems in Neuro-Developmental Handicap: A Team Approach." *Archives of Disease in Childhood*, Vol. 69, 1993, pp. 609-613.

Morris, S.E. and Klein, M.D. *Pre-Feeding Skills: A Comprehensive Resource for Feeding Development*, San Antonio: Therapy Skill Builders, a division of The Psychological Corporation, 1987.

Phelan, P.D. et al. *Pulmonary Complications of Inhalation in Respiratory Illness in Children*. Oxford: Blackwell, 1990, pp. 234-249.

Rosenthal, S. et al. (eds.) *Dysphagia and the Child with Developmental Disabilities: Medical, Clinical, and Family Interventions*, San Diego: Singular Publishing Group, Inc., 1995.

Tuchman, D. and Walter, R. *Disorders of Feeding and Swallowing in Infants and Children: Pathophysiology, Diagnosis, and Treatment*, San Diego: Singular Publishing Group, Inc., 1994.

Wolf, L.P. and Glass, R.P. *Feeding and Swallowing Disorders in Infancy: Assessment and Management*, San Antonio: Therapy Skill Builders, a division of The Psychological Corporation, 1992.

GERD

Booth, I.W. "Silent Gastroesophageal Reflux: How much do we miss?" *Archives of Disease in Childhood*, Vol. 67, 1992, pp. 1325-1327.

Herbst, J.J. "Gastroesophageal Reflux." *The Journal of Pediatrics*, Vol. 98, 1981, pp. 859-870.

Mascarenhas, M.R. and Dadhania, J. "Gastrointestinal Problems." In Rosenthal, S., et al. (eds.) *Dysphagia and the Child with Developmental Disabilities: Medical, Clinical, and Family Interventions*, San Diego: Singular Publishing Group, Inc., 1995, pp. 267-270.

Nielson, D.W. et al. "Stridor and Gastroesophageal Reflux in Infants." *Pediatrics*, Vol. 85, 1990, pp. 1034-1039.

Orenstein, S.R. and Orenstein, D.M. "Gastroesophageal Reflux and Respiratory Disease in Children." *The Journal of Pediatrics*, Vol. 112, 1988, pp. 847-858.

Rossi, T. "Pediatric Gastroenterology." In Arvedson, J. and Brodsky, L. (eds.) *Pediatric Swallowing and Feeding: Assessment and Management*, San Diego: Singular Publishing Group, Inc., 1993, p. 150.

See, C.C. et al. "Gastroesophageal Reflux-Induced Hypoxemia in Infants with Apparent Life Threatening Events (ALTEs). *American Journal of Diseases of Children*, Vol. 143, 1989, pp. 951-954.

Chapter 2: **Medical Disorders**, continued

Head Injury

Clifton, G.L. et al. "Assessment of Nutritional Requirements of Head Injured Patients." *The Journal of Neurosurgery*, Vol. 64, 1986, pp. 895-901.

Epstein, S.M. et al. "Medical Complications of Head Injury." In Cooper, P.R. (ed.) *Head Injury*, Baltimore: Williams and Wilkins, 1987.

Field, L.H. and Weiss, C.J. "Dysphagia with Head Injury." *Brain Injury*, Vol. 3, 1989, pp. 19-26.

Yvilsaker, M. and Logemann, J. "Therapy for Feeding and Swallowing Disorders Following Head Injury." In Yvilsaker, M. (ed.) *Head Injury Rehabilitation: Children and Adolescents*, Boston: College Hill Press, 1995, pp. 195-215.

Yvilsaker, M. and Weinstein, M. "Recovery of Oral Feeding after Pediatric Head Injury." *Journal of Head Trauma Rehabilitation*, Vol. 4, No. 4, 1989, pp. 51-63.

Pierre Robin

Dykes, E.H. et al. "Pierre Robin Syndrome and Pulmonary Hypertension." *Journal of Pediatric Surgery*, Vol. 20, 1985, pp. 49-52.

Sherer, D.M. et al. "Lack of Mandibular Movement Manifested by Absent Fetal Swallowing: A Possible Factor in the Pathogenesis of Micrognathia." *American Journal of Perinatology*, Vol. 12, No. 1, 1995, pp. 30-33.

Shprintzen, R. "Pierre Robin, Micrognathia, and Airway Obstruction: Dependency of Treatment on Accurate Diagnosis." *International Anesthesiology Clinics*, Vol. 26, 1988, pp. 64-71.

Premature Infants

Agnos, S. "Pediatric Swallowing Disorders." Half-day course presented at TFG, Inc. Conference in Nashville, TN, 1998.

American Association of Pediatrics Committee on Nutrition (AAPCON). *Pediatric Nutrition Handbook*, 4th ed, Elk Grove Village, IL: American Academy of Pediatrics, 1998.

Bancalari, E. and Gerhardt, D. "Bronchopulmonary Dysplasia." *Pediatric Clinics of North America*, Vol. 33, 1986, pp. 1-23.

Gill, N. et al. "Effect of Non-nutritive Sucking on Behavioral State in Pre-term Infants before Feeding." *Nursing Research*, Vol. 37, No. 6, 1988, pp. 347-356.

Groh-Wargo, S. et al. *"Nutritional Care for High-Risk Newborns."* 2nd ed. Chicago: Bonus Books, Inc., 1994.

Lau, C. and Schanler, R.J. "Oral-Motor Function in the Neonate." *Clinics in Perinatology*, Vol. 23, No. 2, 1996, pp. 161-178.

Morris, S.E. and Klein, M.D. *Pre-Feeding Skills: A Comprehensive Resource for Feeding Development*. San Antonio: Therapy Skill Builders, a division of The Psychological Corporation, 1987.

Chapter 2: Medical Disorders, continued

Pickler, R. et al. "The Effect of Non-nutritive Sucking on Bottle-Feeding Stress in Preterm Infants." *Journal of Obstetrics, Gynecological, and Neonatal Nursing*, Vol. 22, No. 3, 1993, pp. 230-234.

Pridham, K.F. et al. "Nipple Feeding for Pre-term Infants with Bronchopulmonary Dysplasia." *Journal of Obstetrics, Gynecological, and Neonatal Nursing*, Vol. 22, No. 2, 1993, pp. 147-155.

Redshaw, M. et al. *Born Too Early*, New York: Oxford University Press, 1985.

Saint-Anne Dargassies, S. *Neurological Development in Full-term and Premature Neonate*, New York: Excerpta Medica, 1977.

Shaker, C. "Nipple Feeding Pre-term Infants: A Different Perspective." *Neonatal Network*, Vol. 8, No. 5, 1990, pp. 9-17.

Singer, I.E. et al. "Feeding Interactions in Infants with Very Low Birth Weight and Bronchopulmonary Dysplasia." *Developmental and Behavioral Pediatrics*, Vol. 17, 1996, pp. 69-76.

Updike, C. et al. "Positional Support for Premature Infants." *American Journal of Occupational Therapy*, Vol. 40, No. 10, 1986, pp. 712-715.

Wolf, L.P. and Glass, R.P. *Feeding and Swallowing Disorders in Infancy: Assessment and Management*, San Antonio: Therapy Skill Builders, a division of The Psychological Corporation, 1992.

Wolff, P. "The Serial Organization of Sucking in Young Infants." *Pediatrics*, Vol. 42, 1968, pp. 943-956.

Chapter 3: Clinical Evaluation of Infants and Children

Arvedson (1993) points out that in the assessment of infants and children with feeding disorders it is important to consider:

- oral-motor development
- ability to maintain nutrition and hydration
- relationship and interaction between the caregiver and the child
- medical and/or neurological problems affecting the child

Oral-Motor Development

Oral-motor skills are essential for the child to achieve adequate abilities for eating and drinking by mouth. Depending on the age of the child, you may be able to assess oral-motor skills in isolated movements and during feeding or may be able to assess only during feeding. In order to adequately assess feeding skills in infants and children, it is crucial to understand how these skills develop normally. Information, such as that provided in Chapter 1, must serve as a basis for any assessment of feeding and swallowing skills.

Adequacy of Foods for Nutrition and Hydration

It is important to consult with a clinical nutrition specialist (e.g., Registered Dietitian) concerning the nutritional needs of the infants and children you are assessing for swallowing difficulties. They can provide specific information concerning the child's nutritional status and growth needs. Using only weight gain as an indicator of growth is misleading, especially in a very sick premature infant. The infant's balance of fluids can change very rapidly and alter his body weight (Marx, 1986). If the child is growing appropriately, changes should occur in all body components and not just in weight gain. In other words, the child needs to be growing in skeletal, brain, and fat components.

Caregiver-Child Relationship

The relationship between the child and the child's primary feeder is crucial. Children with oral-motor difficulties may require more time for safe feeding. This can lead to frustration on the feeder's part if she fails to understand that the child needs some compensation during the feeding session, such as changing position, preparing special foods, etc. The feeder may hurry through the feeding. Mathison et al. (1989) found that inner-city children at approximately one year of age with oral-motor dysfunction and non-organic failure to thrive were fed in an average of 8.5 minutes compared to a control group who were fed in an average of 21.1 minutes. They concluded that this suggested an inability of the mothers to accommodate the needs of their children. Other authors agreed that a negative behavioral interaction during feeding can lead to a failure to thrive.

Medical and Neurological Problems

Chapter 8 describes many problems which can be related to feeding disorders or which can cause feeding disorders. Understanding particular medical conditions

Chapter 3: Clinical Evaluation of Infants and Children, continued

and their treatment is important when working with children with multiple disorders.

Multidisciplinary Assessment of Feeding

Many different healthcare professionals may be involved in the assessment of an infant or a child with a feeding disorder. The child's neonatologist or pediatrician is typically the first professional who notices the problem, or to whom the problem is reported. Arvedson (1993) lists the most common criteria for referral of infants and children for an interdisciplinary team assessment. These include:

- sucking and swallowing incoordination
- weak suck
- breathing disruptions or apnea during feeding
- excessive gagging or recurrent coughing during feeding
- new onset of feeding difficulty
- diagnosis of disorders typically associated with dysphagia or failure to thrive
- severe irritability or behavior problems during feeding
- history of recurrent pneumonia and feeding difficulty
- concern for possible aspiration during feeding
- lethargy or decreased arousal during feeding
- feeding periods longer than 30-40 minutes
- unexplained food refusal and failure to thrive
- vomiting
- nasal regurgitation
- increased drooling

Individual professionals can function as an informal team, even if they do not work at the same facility. The professionals involved must communicate their findings to each other and discuss a coordinated approach to treatment. Bryan & Pressman (1995) describe a structured disciplinary diagnostic pediatric dysphagia team. Some of the professionals who may be involved include a general medical practitioner or pediatrician, the feeding specialist (most often a speech-language pathologist [SLP], but in some instances may be an occupational therapist), physical therapist, nurse, and dietitian. Other medical specialties involved may include a pediatric radiologist, a pediatric gastroenterologist, a pediatric pulmonologist, a pediatric otolaryngologist, and a pediatric nutritionist. The caregiver is also a part of the team.

The SLP assesses the child's functional ability to eat safely. This includes an assessment of such things as structural abnormalities, body tone, oral-motor skills, interaction between the caregiver and the child, oral and pharyngeal phases of the swallow, etc. Occupational therapy may assess oral-motor tone, body tone, movement, and in older children, the ability to self-feed. Physical therapy can provide needed information on the child's overall body posture, tone, and movement patterns. A gastroenterologist may see a child who has a history of vomiting or other gastro-intestinal (GI) problems. If the child consistently has

Chapter 3: Clinical Evaluation of Infants and Children, continued

upper respiratory infections and breathing difficulties, the child may see a pulmonologist and/or an allergist. A neurologist will see a child suspected of having a neurological basis for the swallowing disorder. An otolaryngologist may be needed to assess structural abnormalities of the child's mouth and throat.

Who makes most referrals for dysphagia evaluation? Morris (1979) questioned 150 families of infants 4-24 months of age who were being seen for feeding disorders. Seventy-three percent of parents had identified a feeding problem by the time their child was 8 months old. Sixty percent had discussed their concerns with their pediatricians and asked for help with the feeding problems, but only 36% of the families who spoke to their physicians were referred for feeding evaluations. Morris found that the majority were told it was too early to know if the infant had a feeding problem. Although this data is over 20 years old, one might suspect the same situation exists today.

Differences in Adults and Children

Assessing infants and children with feeding problems is different from assessing adults with dysphagia in several ways:

- The anatomy and physiology of these two populations is distinctly different.

- Because the child is growing and changing, the feeding and swallowing function is much more dynamic than it is with an adult. Lefton-Grief (1994) points out that an infant's feeding and swallowing behaviors are continually changing to adapt to his dynamic system.

- The infant or child cannot state he is having trouble swallowing. Dysphagia may not be discovered until it compromises respiratory status, growth, or causes the child to exhibit negative behaviors when presented with food.

- The infant or child is not able to describe the kind of difficulty he is having with feeding. This information often comes from a caregiver who describes what she has observed.

- There is more often a relationship between symptoms in the esophageal and pharyngeal phases in children than adults. When performing a videofluoroscopic evaluation of swallowing in adults, we certainly consider the relationship of esophageal phase disorders to pharyngeal phase disorders. However, Donner (1986) points out that in infants, "Dysphagia . . . is a symptom of disease that may be affecting any part of the swallowing tract from the mouth to the stomach."

Chapter 3: Clinical Evaluation of Infants and Children, continued

- There is a more direct relationship between a child's body posture/tone, ability to move, and ability to eat and swallow than with an adult.

Completing the Feeding Assessment

Ask the caregiver to bring foods the child normally eats and a familiar bib. Also ask the caregiver to bring along the bottle, cup, and other utensils the child usually uses. You will also want to create a feeding kit with a variety of nipples, bottles, spoons, cups, etc. (See Chapter 11). The kit should also contain a variety of food types.

Feeding Evaluation Kit		
Things Caregiver Brings from Home	**Utensils**	**Food and Drink**
bottle cup with lid plate spoon bowl a bib the child is used to wearing small amounts of food the child particularly likes	a variety of cups (e.g., TumbleMates*, Spill Proof**, Pooh Trainer Cup*) plate bowl a variety of spoons (e.g., plastic, metal, Soft Bite Spoons*, Feeding Spoons***) fork straws	cold cereal milk (to add to cereal) soft fruit in juice (e.g., canned peaches) brown bread (e.g., wheat) white bread mashed potato or hot cereal or something that can be heated crackers pudding peanut butter raisins ice cream or sherbet juice iced water

*The First Years
**Playtex
***Gerber

This book includes two separate assessment tools. The first assessment is designed for infants 0-4 months of age (pages 81-83). The cut-off at 4 months of age is used because children younger than 4 months only take nutrition from a bottle and/or breast. At 4-6 months of age, children begin to transition to some cereals and pureed foods, and a cup may be introduced. For that reason, a separate pediatric feeding evaluation for children 4 months and older is included (pages 102-104). Instructions for completing the infant feeding evaluation begin below and continue to page 77. Instructions for completing the pediatric feeding evaluation are on pages 88-98. Completed evaluations and case histories are provided as examples on the pages preceding each assessment (e.g., the example infant feeding evaluation comes directly before the blank infant feeding evaluation).

Chapter 3: Clinical Evaluation of Infants and Children, continued

Obtaining Case History Information

Two separate case histories are included: one for 0-4 months (pages 86-87) and one for 4 months and older (pages 109-112). You may ask the caregiver to complete the case history or you can use it as an interview tool.

Instructions for Completing the Infant Feeding Evaluation (0-4 Months)

History/Background

Date of Birth/ Weeks Gestation/ Adjusted Age

If you are evaluating a premature infant, it is important to assess him at an adjusted age. Normal gestation is 38-40 weeks of age, with 40 considered average. Therefore, if the child was born at less than full gestation, you must adjust their age. For example, a child born on 8-01-98 at 32 weeks gestation is 8 weeks premature. You assess the child on 12-8-98. Chronological age is 18 weeks. Adjusted age is 10 weeks (adjusted age is from 40 weeks gestation date, which for this child would have been 9-26-98, to date of assessment [12-8-98]). In this example, the infant would be developmentally considered 10 weeks old. These adjustments continue until the child is 2 years old.

It is reported that premature infants can coordinate sucking and swallowing at 32 weeks and that feeding can be introduced between 32 and 34 weeks (Klaus & Fanaroff, 1978). However, most studies indicate children will feed more adequately if oral feeding is not begun until 34-35 weeks gestation (Brake et al., 1988).

Medical History

This history can be obtained from the medical record and supplemented by information obtained through caregiver interview. It is important to derive information about the following and include it in the infant's medical history:

- any problems experienced prenatally such as exposure to drug or alcohol abuse, maternal infection, radiation, toxemia, bleeding, or polyhydramnios (i.e., excessive amniotic fluid)

- perinatal problems such as a possible hypoxic event at birth, trauma at delivery, intubation, cardiac status, surfactant therapy (i.e., surfactant is a substance in the lungs to help keep the alveoli inflated)

Chapter 3: Clinical Evaluation of Infants and Children, continued

- Apgar scores*
- genetic problems
- overall development pattern
- gastrointestinal problems
- respiratory problems
- formal medical diagnoses or conditions
- related surgical procedures
- medications that may affect child's level of alertness or swallowing skills
- current methods for nutrition and hydration
- current weight, usually given in grams for premature infants
- amount of tube feedings (infant may be full, and not interested in taking anything by mouth)
- any previous evaluations
- family history of any similar problems (e.g., cleft palate or craniofacial problems)

*The Apgar scale is used to make a quick and thorough examination of a neonate's response to the birth process and immediate adaptation to life outside the uterus. The infant is usually rated at 60 seconds after birth and at 5 minutes after birth. The infant is rated on heart rate, respiratory effort, muscle tone, irritability, and color on a scale of 0 through 10.

Sleep Patterns   Pre-term infants often require more sleep than full-term babies. They are not as readily available for interaction because it is more difficult to wake them up. Sick infants seem to have a difficult time regulating their biological rhythms regarding wakefulness, and therefore, may sleep more often and for longer periods of time.

Feeding Patterns   Find out how much the infant eats, how long it takes for the infant to eat, and how often the infant eats.

Feeding Concerns Reported   List the specific problems that the referring medical personnel and/or caregiver describe as the reasons the infant was referred. These might include any of the following:

Chapter 3: Clinical Evaluation of Infants and Children, *continued*

- sucking and swallowing incoordination
- weak suck
- breathing disruptions or apnea during feeding
- excessive gagging or recurrent coughing during feeding
- new onset of feeding difficulty
- diagnosis of disorders typically associated with dysphagia or failure to thrive
- severe irritability or behavior problems during feeding
- history of recurrent pneumonia and feeding difficulty
- concern for possible aspiration during feeds
- lethargy or decreased arousal during feeds
- feeding periods longer than 30-40 minutes
- unexplained food refusal and failure to thrive
- vomiting
- nasal regurgitation
- increased drooling

Wolf and Glass (1992) provide a very helpful table which clusters similar symptoms that suggest the need for more careful assessment in a certain area. (See Appendix 3-A, page 113.)

Infant's State

It is important to note the state the infant is in before you begin your interaction, any changes that occur in the infant's state during interaction, and the infant's state after you finish feeding the infant and place the infant back in the crib. Select the state that best describes the baby at each point in the interaction (Brazelton, 1984).

> State 1: Deep Sleep
> The baby has a regular respiratory pattern with eyes closed and no eye movement.

Chapter 3: Clinical Evaluation of Infants and Children, continued

State 2: Light Sleep
The infant's eyes are closed, but rapid eye movements may be noted beneath the lids and the infant may open her eyes occasionally. Respirations are irregular and sucking movements may be seen.

State 3: Drowsy or Semi-dozing
The child's eyes are open, but dull with eyelids fluttering. The child may look dazed.

State 4: Quiet Alert
The infant is focused on stimulus with a bright look.

State 5: Active Alert
The infant exhibits considerable motor activity with thrusting of the extremities and may have brief fussy periods.

State 6: Crying
The infant is crying intensely and it is difficult to get the child to stop.

Physiologic Function

The infants you evaluate between the ages of 0-4 months will probably be in the Neonatal Intensive Care Unit, in another hospital unit, or at home. Wherever the infants are, they will probably be on many monitors. Nursing personnel can help you observe the child's heart rate and respiratory rate on monitors and oxygen saturation level on a pulse oximeter. Note the baseline ratings before you begin interacting with the infant, any changes during the interaction, and the rates after the child has quieted and you have returned him to his crib.

Heart rate: If the child is hooked up to a cardiac/respiratory monitor, it will provide an average numeric value. It will typically sound an alarm if the child goes beyond an upper or lower limit. Be sure the baseline heart rate value is taken when the baby is awake and quiet.

Full-term neonates typically have a heart rate between 120-140 beats per minute, though rates between 70 and 170 may be considered acceptable (Chow et al., 1984). Heart rates are lower during sleep and higher with activity. During feeding, the heartbeat may increase 10 beats a minute over baseline value. Resting heart rate is generally higher in premature infants than in full-term

Chapter 3: Clinical Evaluation of Infants and Children, continued

neonates, with a baseline being reported at 160-180 beats per minute (Chow et al., 1984).

Changes in heart rate may include tachycardia (i.e., elevated heart rate) or bradycardia (i.e., a drop in heart rate below 90-100 beats per minute). Bradycardia is a serious problem that may be life threatening. It is necessary to change whatever you are doing when feeding the infant to eliminate a drop in heart rate. Bradycardia may occur if the infant is aspirating or experiencing a laryngospasm causing apnea, which brings on a decrease in oxygen saturation, which brings on the bradycardia.

Respiratory Rate: Typical newborns are thought to have respiratory rates between 30-60 breaths a minute (Krane, 1986). Respiratory rates tend to be highest when infants are awake and lowest when asleep. If a high respiratory rate occurs during feeding, consult with nursing staff to determine how high it can go before you should stop your feeding assessment. Remember that infants at this age sequence one suck to one swallow (takes about 1 second) and each suck-swallow is paired by an apneic period while the child stops breathing. This means that the child's respiratory rate is probably going to be 40-50 breaths per minute while swallowing.

An infant may be identified as a mouth breather when the mouth is open only because he does not have the necessary sensory cues or muscle tone to help him maintain closure. Nelson & DeBeenabib (1991) indicate that this can be checked by closing the infant's jaw and lips and observing whether the infant tries to push air through his lips or continues breathing normally through his nose.

Oxygen Saturation (SaO^2): Oxygen saturation is the amount of oxygen in the blood. It is expressed as a percent of 100. In most conditions, normal infants have oxygen saturation above 95 percent and pre-term babies at or above 90 percent. Any rate below 90 percent indicates some degree of hypoxia.

Structure/Function

Structural Deformities Check the medical record to see if the child has any of the following:

Chapter 3: Clinical Evaluation of Infants and Children, *continued*

- tracheomalacia (i.e., softening of the cartilages in the trachea)

- esophageal atresia

- TE fistula: If the infant has a TE fistula, you will not be able to present any food during your assessment because anything the child swallows will travel through the TE fistula into the trachea and the lungs

- subglottic stenosis

Trunk Take off the infant's shirt to observe his trunk. Note tone in the trunk. At the same time, observe respiratory patterns. (See page 71.)

Jaw Observe the jaw at rest to see if there is any asymmetry. Watch the infant open his jaw. Notice if there is a thrust or asymmetry on opening.

Lips Observe the infant's lips at rest to see if there is any asymmetry.

Tongue Observe the infant's tongue at rest for asymmetry. Also look at the frenum. Make sure there is no restriction of the frenum. The tongue should move easily past the lips.

Cheeks Observe the tone of the cheeks at rest.

Palate The hard palate assists with stability of the nipple and helps the tongue compress the nipple.

Determine if the infant has a reported cleft of the hard palate. This might be a unilateral cleft, a bilateral cleft, or a sub-mucous cleft. A unilateral or bilateral cleft of the hard palate is almost certain to cause swallowing difficulties. (See Chapter 2.) Clefts of the soft palate may also cause feeding difficulties as the child may have difficulty obtaining velopharyngeal closure or closure of the palate against the base of the tongue for good oral pressure for sucking. If an infant has had a prolonged oro-tracheal intubation, the tube may have caused a groove to form in the middle of the hard palate and alveolar ridge. This can interfere with sucking.

Chapter 3: Clinical Evaluation of Infants and Children, *continued*

Gums	Some medications (e.g., seizure medications) can cause swelling in the gums. If the mouth is sore, the infant is less likely to want to eat.
Respiration	Remove the infant's shirt and observe if the infant appears to be breathing adequately, showing some shallow breathing, showing extreme movement of the belly for belly breathing, showing reverse breathing (thoracic musculature appears to be breathing in while abdominal muscles are breathing out), or showing thoracic breathing in which the upper chest area moves excessively during breathing.
Hypersensitivity	Note the infant's reaction to being touched on the face or in the mouth. Hypersensitivity may interfere with adequate feeding.

Non-Nutritive Sucking Observation

Burst cycles	Non-nutritive sucking (as well as nutritive sucking) occurs in bursts, followed by pauses. Determine the pattern the infant is exhibiting. How many sucks does the infant exhibit in a burst before pausing?
Endurance deficits	Make a subjective judgment about the infant's ability to continue non-nutritive sucking for a period of time. Non-nutritive sucking is faster that nutritive sucking. The child should be sucking approximately two sucks per second and typically for a burst of 7-8 sucks, with a pause of 6-7 seconds in between (Wolff, 1968). If the infant seems to wear out very quickly and stops non-nutritive sucking, this might be judged as a severe deficit in endurance.
Closure of lips on finger/nipple	After you put the glove on, get it wet before you put your finger in the infant's mouth as the infant may accept it more easily. These infants have had many medical procedures performed about the face and in the mouth and recognize the feel of a gloved finger (Conley and Hale, 1997). See if the infant obtains lip closure.
Tongue cup/ groove and suck strength	Place your finger, pad down, in the mouth. Make a judgment about how well the tongue cups/grooves and the strength of the suck.
Cardiopulmonary changes	Note any change in cardiac status, respiratory status, and pattern of breathing. A coordinated pattern of 6-8 sucks followed by a swallow and a rest period to breathe should be noted. If not observed, check "incoordinated suck/swallow/breathe."

Chapter 3: Clinical Evaluation of Infants and Children, continued

---

Also note if the infant engages in "catch-up" breathing. Catch-up breathing occurs when the infant stops for a much longer period of time to breathe before returning to non-nutritive sucking. You also might notice short breaths/pants during the pauses rather than calm, easy breathing.

Nutritive Sucking Observation

Normal Reflexes

rooting: Note whether the infant exhibits a rooting reflex when stimulated at the right, left, or at midline of lips. An absent or diminished reflex may indicate poor tactile sensation or integration of tactile stimuli (Wolf and Glass, 1992). If the infant exhibits excessive rooting, he may have hypersensitivity or a lack of inhibition. Rooting should disappear between 3-6 months.

suckle-swallow: Touch your finger or the nipple lightly to the infant's lips or tongue to see if suckling begins. If so, the finger or nipple will be drawn into the mouth and active suckling will be observed. If you get no response initially, evaluate again. The infant may not have been alert enough or may not have been hungry. If a reduced suckling reflex or absent suckling reflex is consistently found, it usually indicates a neurological disorder (Wolf and Glass, 1992).

Abnormal Reflexes

Do not specifically elicit abnormal reflexes. Observe for the occurrence of any of these during feeding.

tonic bite: strong closure of the jaw when teeth or gums are stimulated. It may be difficult for the infant to release the bite.

jaw thrust: strong downward extension of the lower jaw. The jaw may appear to be stuck open.

tongue retraction: strong pulling back of the tongue into the hypopharynx. The tip of the tongue may be held against the hard palate.

tongue thrust: forceful protrusion of the tongue from the mouth

overactive gag: gag reflex stimulated in front of mouth

Chapter 3: Clinical Evaluation of Infants and Children, *continued*

Feeding Position Note how the caregiver holds the infant while feeding. Is the infant lying on his back with his head elevated just a bit or is the whole body slightly elevated? Is the infant lying on his side or on his belly?

Infants with tracheomalacia, laryngomalacia, or laryngo-tracheomalacia (i.e., softening of the cartilages in the trachea, larynx, or both) may do better in a sidelying position because gravity reduces the effect of the collapsed airway.

Bottle/Breast

Note if the evaluation is completed with infant using bottle or breast.

Suck/Swallow/Breathe Pattern In young infants, the typical pattern is one suck, one swallow, and one pause for breathing. That is, the child sucks once to draw fluid into the mouth, stops breathing to swallow the fluid, and then breathes. In older infants, two or three sucks may occur per swallow.

Burst cycles With nutritive sucking, an infant usually shows an initial continuous sucking burst for at least the first 30 seconds, and sometimes as much as 60-80 seconds. That means that during the first minute, the infant is showing a suck/swallow/breathe pattern continuing for up to 60-80 seconds before pausing to rest. As the infant becomes satiated, the infant then has fewer sucks in each burst and longer pauses (Mathew et al., 1985; Shivpuri et al., 1983). By the end of a feeding, the infant may be only showing two to three sucks in a burst.

Fluid expression This is a subjective judgment. With bottle feeding, bubbles should be observed with each swallow. You have to judge whether the infant is getting enough with each suck. A problem in this area may be indicated by an infant who sucks three or four times before swallowing. This probably means that the infant is having to work too hard to express any of the fluid.

Anterior loss Some loss around a nipple is normal for an infant. Mark if there is excessive loss.

Endurance Endurance is related to the amount of liquid consumed and the length of time it takes an infant to consume the liquid. Does the infant stay alert throughout feeding without appearing fatigued? Each feeding should take no longer than 20 minutes.

Chapter 3: Clinical Evaluation of Infants and Children, *continued*

Does the infant consume an adequate amount before becoming fatigued? Infants up to one month of age should take 2-6 ounces before showing shorter bursts and less interest in sucking. By the time infants are three months of age, they should be taking 7-8 ounces at each feeding.

Amount consumed   birth to 1 month: 2-6 ounces (56-168cc) during each of 6 or more feedings a day

3 months: 7-8 ounces during each of 4-6 feedings a day

Response to Feeding

Type of Distress   An infant has a variety of ways to indicate he is having difficulty with the feeding. Some of these responses might be considered moderate and are listed in the chart under the header "Moderate."

Other symptoms are more major: breath holding, gagging, choking, changes in respiratory pattern, etc. Note any of these responses, but also respond to these distress signals by making changes. (See Chapter 6.)

Pharyngeal Symptoms

Note any pharyngeal symptoms. As in the adult population, children can also be silent aspirators. Arvedson et al. (1992) reviewed videofluroscopic evaluations of 186 children. Aspiration was found in 48 of the children. The aspiration was silent in 45 of the 48.

Response to Compensations

If an infant is having difficulty during the assessment, you want to try some techniques to see if you can improve the child's performance. As in most assessments performed by SLPs, there is a component of stimulability testing which occurs. A more detailed description of these techniques is provided in Chapter 5 and Chapter 6. A short description is given here. On any compensation that you attempt, note the infant's response.

Support to lips   If the infant is having excessive anterior loss, provide a little support at the corners of the lips to help the infant get better closure.

Chapter 3: Clinical Evaluation of Infants and Children, continued

External jaw support Excessive anterior loss may also be caused by reduced jaw control. Place a finger lightly under the infant's chin to provide some support.

External cheek support Sometimes the infant can't get good suction because of decreased tone in the cheeks. Using your thumb and middle finger on the hand which is holding the bottle, provide some support to the cheeks to help the infant achieve some stability in his suck.

Change in posture You might try a more flexed pattern with shoulders pulled forward and chin tucked to provide a little better airway protection. You might also try sidelying for the infant with poor head control.

External pacing External pacing may be accomplished by pulling the nipple away or tipping the bottle so there is no fluid in the nipple. This technique is helpful for infants who seem to have a hard time organizing their suck/swallow/breathe pattern.

Calming/ organizing/ alerting A variety of calming/organizing/alerting techniques are described in detail in Chapter 6. If an infant is not in an appropriate state during the feeding, stop, use these techniques, and then try to continue the assessment.

Establish non-nutritive suck If an infant is having difficulty coordinating suck/swallow/breathe when you present the bottle, stop and return to a non-nutritive suck on a pacifier or finger. This may help the infant organize the suck/swallow/breathe pattern. You can then return to the assessment with nutritive sucking. Frequent breaks for burping may be needed and may even facilitate endurance. Use the burping break to introduce non-nutritive sucking to help the infant organize (Comrie and Helm, 1997).

Provide oral stimulation For the infant who fails to latch on (i.e., achieve tight closure with lips and tongue), providing some oral stimulation may increase the infant's readiness for feeding.

Negative resistance Comrie and Helm (1997) describe a technique to use with infants who use a biting pattern rather than a sucking pattern or for infants who have an inefficient and rapid sucking pattern. Provide timed negative resistance during the infant's attempts to suck. As the infant pulls in the nipple slightly during sucking, gently tug on the nipple to create a stronger suck. If the technique is successful, longer and larger streams of bubbles should be observed. Never

Chapter 3: Clinical Evaluation of Infants and Children, continued

pull the nipple so hard that it comes out of the infant's mouth or breaks the suction seal. This negative resistance may also facilitate organization and conserve energy. Comrie and Helm advise using this with firm jaw support.

Change in nipple   Avoid changing nipples numerous times during an assessment as this will only confuse the child. If one nipple seems very inappropriate (see Chapter 11), stop and give the infant a rest and then continue with a different type of nipple. Remember that the flow rate of the nipple can change breathing (Shivpuri et al., 1983). Mathew (1991) noted a decrease in the amount of breathing done in one minute with preemies using a high-flow nipple (preemie nipples are high-flow nipples). Mathew indicated that this may suggest that high-flow nipples yield a greater ventilatory compromise.

Thicken liquids   Slightly thickening the liquids helps children who have poor motor control. It also helps infants with significant gastroesophageal reflux and projectile vomiting.

Change in utensils   Note if a different type of bottle (e.g., angle-neck) was helpful.

Recommendations

Getting the infant in the appropriate state   Often infants need to be calmed/organized or alerted before feeding. These techniques are described in detail in Chapter 6. List the techniques you used and found helpful to guide the child to the appropriate state.

Position the infant   Provide recommendations about the best way to position the infant for feeding.

Use bottle/ nipple/pacifier   Describe the kind of pacifier and nipple you found to be most successful with the infant. Most often you want to use the same shape pacifier nipple as you do on the bottle.

Frequency of feeding/ schedule   Considerations here include how quickly the infant fatigues. If the infant wears out and cannot finish the feeding, more frequent, shorter feedings may be indicated. Typical infants at birth to one month of age take six or more feedings a day. By three months, this is reduced to 4-6 feedings a day. Consult with the infant's pediatrician or neonatologist and nursing staff to help determine the appropriate feeding schedule.

Chapter 3: Clinical Evaluation of Infants and Children, continued

Environment Note the environment which seemed the most appropriate. The infant may need a calm environment without much background noise or movement in order to maintain an organized state. The infant may also respond to rocking or to the use of music. For some infants, rocking or music tends to decrease their level of alertness.

Stress signals Note any stress signals the infant exhibits which you recorded under *Response to Feeding*. Caregivers are not always aware that these kinds of movements indicate stress. Indicate how the feeder should respond to the stress signals.

Temperature of formula Note whether the infant responded better to warm or cold temperatures.

Caloric value Consult with dietitian and nursing staff concerning the kind of feeding needed.

Pacing Note if the infant seemed to need breaks.

Further evaluation Note if the infant needs any further diagnostic evaluations or consultations.

Chapter 3: Clinical Evaluation of Infants and Children, continued

Example Infant Feeding Evaluation (0-4 months)

Name: __Serena__   Patient #: _____   Date of Eval.: __10-30-98__

DOB: __9-25-98__   Weeks Gestation/Adjusted Age: __32 wks./still 3 wks. younger than normal gestation__

Medical History: __born prematurely @ 32 weeks; intubated w/ventilatory support for 3 weeks; hypotonic__

Current Weight: __1700 grams__   Amount Tube Feeding: __40 cc every 3 hours__   MD: __P. Mature__

Sleep Patterns: __awake only for feedings & shortly before__

Feeding Patterns: __NG tube - began to try oral feedings 2 weeks ago__

Feeding Concerns Reported: __takes very little by mouth, weak suck__

Infant's State	Pre-	During	After
Deep Sleep			
Light Sleep			
Drowsy/Semi-dozing	✔	✔*	
Quiet Alert			
Active Alert			
Crying			

Physiologic Function	Pre-	During	After
Heart Rate	160	170	160
Respiratory Rate	35	45	35
SaO²	90	80	89

* need to keep alerting

Structure/Function

Structural Deformities
☐ tracheomalacia
☐ esophageal atresia
☐ TE fistula
☐ subglottic stenosis

Trunk
☑ tone __low__

Jaw
☐ asymmetry at rest
☐ opening
___ thrust
___ asymmetry

Lips
☐ asymmetric at rest

Tongue
☐ asymmetric at rest
☐ frenum restricts protrusion

Cheeks
☐ abnormal tone at rest

Palate
☐ cleft hard palate (uni/bi/sub)
☐ cleft soft palate

Gums
☐ swollen/cracked

Respiration
☑ shallow breathing
☐ belly breathing
☐ reverse breathing
☐ thoracic breathing

Hypersensitivity
☐ face
☐ mouth

Non-Nutritive Sucking Observation

Burst cycles: __✔__ 1-5   ____ 5-12   ____ 12-15

Endurance deficits: ____ mild   __✔__ moderate   ____ severe

Closure of lips on finger/nipple: ____ adequate   __✔__ weak

Tongue cupped/grooved: ____ yes   __✔__ no

Suck strength: __✔__ weak   ____ adequate

Cardiopulmonary changes:
__✔__ incoordinated suck/swallow/breathe
__✔__ catch-up breathing
____ short breaths/pants

Comments:
_____
_____
_____
_____

Chapter 3: Clinical Evaluation of Infants and Children, continued

Example Infant Feeding Evaluation (0-4 months), continued

Name: _Serena_

Nutritive Sucking Observation

Normal Reflexes
☐ rooting (R/L/mid)
☑ suckle-swallow

Abnormal Reflexes
☐ tonic bite
☐ jaw thrust
☐ tongue retraction
☐ tongue thrust
☐ overactive gag

Feeding Position
☑ supine with head elevated a bit
☐ prone
☐ sidelying
☐ slightly elevated

Bottle ✔   Breast ____

Suck/Swallow/Breathe pattern
_2-3_ # sucks to swallow

Burst cycles
initial burst: ✔ 30 sec. ____ 45 sec. ____ 60 sec.
____ follows normal pattern of steady decline   ✔ declines much too quickly

Fluid expression
____ good ✔ fair ____ poor

Anterior loss
____ normal ✔ excessive

Endurance
____ adequate ✔ decreased

Amount consumed:
_15cc_ in _30_ minutes

Response to Feeding

Moderate Distress

sighing		increased hypertonicity		startling	
yawning	✔	increased hypotonicity	✔	gasping	
facial grimacing		sneezing		straining	
squirming		sweating		bowel movement	
averting gaze		hiccuping		multiple swallows	
falling asleep		trembling (jaw/limb)			

Major Distress

coughing	✔	color change	
spitting up		respiratory pauses	
gagging		irregular respiration	
choking		arching back	
breath holding		bradycardia	

Chapter 3: Clinical Evaluation of Infants and Children, continued

Example Infant Feeding Evaluation (0-4 months), continued

Name: _Serena_

Pharyngeal Symptoms

☐ congestion ☑ coughing ☐ multiple swallows
☑ changes in breathing ☐ wet breath sounds ☐ wet vocal sounds

Response to Compensations

Support to lips	much less anterior loss
External jaw support	seems to increase strength of closure
External cheek support	
Change in posture (describe)	a little more upright, swaddled, light flexion
External pacing	
pull nipple away	
bottle tipping	calmed her when she choked
Calming/(organizing)/alerting	swaddle w/shoulders forward
Establish non-nutritive suck	
Provide oral stimulation	
lip tap	increases closure - needs throughout feeding
lingual stroke/tap	
Negative resistance	
Change in nipple (describe)	softer red preemie nipple for faster flow - infant got more volume
Thicken liquids	
Change in utensils (describe)	angle-neck bottle easier to use w/flexion
Other (describe)	tap feet to re-alert

Recommendations

Getting infant in appropriate state: _unwrap to cool, then reswaddle_
Position the infant: _upright 70° w/flexion_
Bottle: _angle-neck_   Nipple: _preemie_   Pacifier: _preemie_
Frequency of feeding/schedule: _every 3 hours_   Environment: _lights on, visual stimuli_
Watch for these stress signals: _yawning, coughing_   Respond to stress signals by: _tipping bottle_
Temperature of formula: _warm_   Caloric value: _____   Pacing: _tip bottle every 45-60 secs._
Other: _oral stim as needed during feeding; tap feet to re-alert_
Further evaluation: _consider MBS if these changes do not eliminate coughing_

_____   _____ _____ _____
SLP   Date   Time   Procedure

The Source for Pediatric Dysphagia

Chapter 3: Clinical Evaluation of Infants and Children, *continued*

Infant Feeding Evaluation (0-4 months)

Name: _____ Patient #: _____ Date of Eval.: _____

DOB: _____ Weeks Gestation/Adjusted Age: _____

Medical History: _____
_____

Current Weight: _____ Amount Tube Feeding: _____ MD: _____
Sleep Patterns: _____
Feeding Patterns: _____
Feeding Concerns Reported: _____

Infant's State	Pre-	During	After
Deep Sleep			
Light Sleep			
Drowsy/Semi-dozing			
Quiet Alert			
Active Alert			
Crying			

Physiologic Function	Pre-	During	After
Heart Rate			
Respiratory Rate			
SaO^2			

Structure/Function

Structural Deformities
☐ tracheomalacia
☐ esophageal atresia
☐ TE fistula
☐ subglottic stenosis

Trunk
☐ tone _____

Jaw
☐ asymmetry at rest
☐ opening
___ thrust
___ asymmetry

Lips
☐ asymmetric at rest

Tongue
☐ asymmetric at rest
☐ frenum restricts protrusion

Cheeks
☐ abnormal tone at rest

Palate
☐ cleft hard palate (uni/bi/sub)
☐ cleft soft palate

Gums
☐ swollen/cracked

Respiration
☐ shallow breathing
☐ belly breathing
☐ reverse breathing
☐ thoracic breathing

Hypersensitivity
☐ face
☐ mouth

Non-Nutritive Sucking Observation

Burst cycles: ____ 1-5 ____ 5-12 ____ 12-15

Endurance deficits: ____ mild ____ moderate
____ severe

Closure of lips on finger/nipple:
____ adequate ____ weak

Tongue cupped/grooved: ____ yes ____ no

Suck strength: ____ weak ____ adequate

Cardiopulmonary changes:
____ incoordinated suck/swallow/breathe
____ catch-up breathing
____ short breaths/pants

Comments:
_____
_____
_____
_____

The Source for Pediatric Dysphagia

Chapter 3: Clinical Evaluation of Infants and Children, continued

Infant Feeding Evaluation (0-4 months), continued

Name: _____

Nutritive Sucking Observation

Normal Reflexes	**Abnormal Reflexes**	**Feeding Position**
☐ rooting (R/L/mid)	☐ tonic bite	☐ supine with head elevated a bit
☐ suckle-swallow	☐ jaw thrust	☐ prone
	☐ tongue retraction	☐ sidelying
	☐ tongue thrust	☐ slightly elevated
	☐ overactive gag	

Bottle _____   **Breast** _____

Suck/Swallow/Breathe pattern
_____ # sucks to swallow

Burst cycles
initial burst: _____ 30 sec. _____ 45 sec. _____ 60 sec.
_____ follows normal pattern of steady decline   _____ declines much too quickly

Fluid expression
_____ good _____ fair _____ poor

Anterior loss
_____ normal _____ excessive

Endurance
_____ adequate _____ decreased

Amount consumed:
_____ in _____ minutes

Response to Feeding

sighing	
yawning	
facial grimacing	
squirming	
averting gaze	
falling asleep	

Moderate Distress

increased hypertonicity	
increased hypotonicity	
sneezing	
sweating	
hiccuping	
trembling (jaw/limb)	

startling	
gasping	
straining	
bowel movement	
multiple swallows	

Major Distress

coughing	
spitting up	
gagging	
choking	
breath holding	

color change	
respiratory pauses	
irregular respiration	
arching back	
bradycardia	

The Source for Pediatric Dysphagia

Chapter 3: Clinical Evaluation of Infants and Children, continued

Infant Feeding Evaluation (0-4 months), continued

Name: _____

Pharyngeal Symptoms

☐ congestion   ☐ coughing   ☐ multiple swallows
☐ changes in breathing   ☐ wet breath sounds   ☐ wet vocal sounds

Response to Compensations

Support to lips	
External jaw support	
External cheek support	
Change in posture (describe)	
External pacing	
pull nipple away	
bottle tipping	
Calming/organizing/alerting	
Establish non-nutritive suck	
Provide oral stimulation	
lip tap	
lingual stroke/tap	
Negative resistance	
Change in nipple (describe)	
Thicken liquids	
Change in utensils (describe)	
Other (describe)	

Recommendations

Getting infant in appropriate state: _____
Position the infant: _____
Bottle: _____ Nipple: _____ Pacifier: _____
Frequency of feeding/schedule: _____ Environment: _____
Watch for these stress signals: _____ Respond to stress signals by: _____
Temperature of formula: _____ Caloric value: _____ Pacing: _____
Other: _____
Further evaluation: _____

_____   _____   _____   _____
SLP   Date   Time   Procedure

The Source for Pediatric Dysphagia

Chapter 3: Clinical Evaluation of Infants and Children, continued

Example Case History/Interview Form for Infants with Feeding Problems (0-4 months)

Name: __Serena__ Date of Eval.: __10-30-98__

DOB: __9-25-98__ Age: __5 weeks__

Address: _____

Caregiver(s): __Mom__

Home phone: _____ Work phone: _____

Primary care physician: __P. Mature__

Other physicians treating child: __lung doctor__

Why is your child being seen for a feeding evaluation? __will not eat enough to get tube out__

Medical History

Has your child had any surgeries? ____ yes __✔__ no

If yes, please list with dates: _____

Has your child ever been hospitalized? __✔__ yes ____ no

If yes, please list reason(s) and date(s): __still in hospital__

Is your child on any medication(s)? __✔__ yes ____ no

If yes, please list: __multivitamins with iron, Theophillin®__

Does your child have any allergies (food or otherwise)? ____ yes __✔__ no

If yes, please list: _____

Birth History

Weight of your child at birth: __1275 grams__

Was your child full-term? ____ yes __✔__ no

If no, how many weeks gestation? __30__

Were there any problems during pregnancy? __✔__ yes ____ no

If yes, please describe: __pre-eclamptic; HTN__

Were there any problems immediately after birth? __✔__ yes ____ no

If yes, please describe: __baby turned blue, had to be put on a breathing machine__

The Source for Pediatric Dysphagia

Chapter 3: Clinical Evaluation of Infants and Children, continued

Example Case History for Infants (0-4 months), continued

Feeding History

Was your child breast-fed? _____ yes __✔__ no

If *yes*, how long? _____ Were there any problems with this (e.g., poor suck, slow to feed)? _____

When was your child first given a bottle? _2 weeks ago_ Were there any problems with this (e.g., poor suck, slow to feed)? _doesn't take much_

How many times a day is your child fed? _7-8_

How is your child positioned when eating (e.g., held by caregiver, swaddled in blanket, held facing caregiver)? _held by me or nurse_

Does your child eat more/less when he/she is at daycare/baby-sitter/grandparents/other? (Please describe.) _n/a_

Does your child receive supplemental (tube) feeding: __✔__ yes _____ no

If *yes*, amount _____ NG: __✔__

rate _____ PEG: _____

PEJ: _____

Bolus (given via syringe several times a day): __✔__

Continuous (connected to pump): _____

How much liquid does your child drink at each meal (approximately)? _5-6 cc_

How long does each meal take? _30-40 minutes_

Person completing form: _____

Date: _12-30-98_

The Source for Pediatric Dysphagia

Chapter 3: Clinical Evaluation of Infants and Children, *continued*

Case History/Interview Form for Infants with Feeding Problems (0-4 months)

Name: _____ Date of Eval.: _____

DOB: _____ Age: _____

Address: _____

Caregiver(s): _____

Home phone: _____ Work phone: _____

Primary care physician: _____

Other physicians treating child: _____

Why is your child being seen for a feeding evaluation? _____

_____

Medical History

Has your child had any surgeries? _____ yes _____ no

If *yes*, please list with dates: _____

_____

Has your child ever been hospitalized? _____ yes _____ no

If *yes*, please list reason(s) and date(s): _____

_____

Is your child on any medication(s)? _____ yes _____ no

If *yes*, please list: _____

Does your child have any allergies (food or otherwise)? _____ yes _____ no

If *yes*, please list: _____

Birth History

Weight of your child at birth: _____

Was your child full-term? _____ yes _____ no

If *no*, how many weeks gestation? _____

Were there any problems during pregnancy? _____ yes _____ no

If *yes*, please describe: _____

Were there any problems immediately after birth? _____ yes _____ no

If *yes*, please describe: _____

The Source for Pediatric Dysphagia

Chapter 3: Clinical Evaluation of Infants and Children, continued

Case History for Infants (0-4 months), continued

Feeding History

Was your child breast-fed? _____ yes _____ no

If *yes*, how long? _____ Were there any problems with this (e.g., poor suck, slow to feed)? _____

When was your child first given a bottle? _____ Were there any problems with this (e.g., poor suck, slow to feed)? _____
_____

How many times a day is your child fed? _____

How is your child positioned when eating (e.g., held by caregiver, swaddled in blanket, held facing caregiver)? _____
_____

Does your child eat more/less when he/she is at daycare/baby-sitter/grandparents/other? (Please describe.) _____
_____

Does your child receive supplemental (tube) feeding: _____ yes _____ no

If *yes*, amount _____ NG: _____
    rate _____ PEG: _____
                              PEJ: _____

Bolus (given via syringe several times a day): _____

Continuous (connected to pump): _____

How much liquid does your child drink at each meal (approximately)? _____

How long does each meal take? _____

Person completing form: _____

Date: _____

Chapter 3: Clinical Evaluation of Infants and Children, *continued*

Instructions for Completing the Pediatric Feeding Evaluation (4 months and older)

Medical History

This history can be obtained from the medical record and supplemented by information obtained through caregiver interview. It is important to derive information about the following and include it in the child's medical history:

- any problems experienced prenatally such as exposure to drug or alcohol abuse, maternal infection, radiation, toxemia, bleeding, or polyhydramnios (i.e., excessive amniotic fluid)

- perinatal problems such as a possible hypoxic event at birth, trauma at delivery, intubation, cardiac status, surfactant therapy (i.e., surfactant is a substance in the lungs to help keep the alveoli inflated)

- Apgar scores*

- genetic problems

- overall development pattern

- gastrointestinal problems

- respiratory problems

- formal medical diagnoses or conditions

- related surgical procedures

- medications that may affect child's level of alertness or swallowing skills

- current methods for nutrition and hydration

- any previous evaluations

- family history of any similar problems (e.g., cleft palate or craniofacial problems)

*The Apgar scale is used to make a quick and thorough examination of a neonate's response to the birth process and immediate adaptation to life outside the uterus. The infant is usually rated at 60 seconds after birth and 5 minutes after birth. The infant is rated on heart rate, respiratory effort, muscle tone, irritability, and color on a scale of 0 through 10.

Chapter 3: Clinical Evaluation of Infants and Children, continued

Feeding Patterns

Find out how much the child eats, how long it takes for the child to eat, and how often the child eats.

Feeding Concerns Reported

List the specific problem(s) that the referring medical personnel and/or caregiver describe as the reason the child was referred. These might include any of the following:

- sucking and swallowing incoordination
- weak suck
- breathing disruptions or apnea during feeding
- excessive gagging or recurrent coughing during feeding
- new onset of feeding difficulty
- diagnosis of disorders typically associated with dysphagia or failure to thrive
- severe irritability or behavior problems during feeding
- history of recurrent pneumonia and feeding difficulty
- concern for possible aspiration during feeds
- lethargy or decreased arousal during feeds
- feeding periods longer than 30 - 40 minutes
- unexplained food refusal and failure to thrive
- vomiting
- nasal regurgitation
- increased drooling

Wolf and Glass (1992) provide a very helpful table which clusters similar symptoms that suggest the need for more careful assessment in a certain area. (See Appendix 3-A, page 113.)

Chapter 3: Clinical Evaluation of Infants and Children, continued

Structure/Function

Depending on the age of the child, you may be able to assess some of these things in isolation by having the child imitate motor movements. Others may need to be observed as the child is lying or sitting.

Contractures   Note if the child has any contractures.

Trunk   Note tone in the trunk. For a child who is sitting independently, see if he is able to lean to one side or the other and flex his trunk (lateral trunk flexion).

From a sitting position, see if the child can turn his entire trunk to reach in one direction or the other (trunk rotation).

Head Control   Note if the child can maintain head at midline or if the head slumps to one side or the other. By 5-7 months, the child should be able to sit independently and maintain head control.

Jaw   Observe the jaw at rest to see if there is any asymmetry. Watch the child open his jaw. Notice if there is a thrust or asymmetry on opening.

Lips   Observe the child's lips at rest to see if there is any asymmetry. Determine if the child is maintaining closure at rest. If the child is old enough, ask the child to imitate lip spreading and lip puckering.

Tongue   Observe the child's tongue at rest for asymmetry. Also look at the frenum. Make sure there is no restriction of the frenum. The tongue should move easily past the lips.

See if the child will imitate tongue protrusion and tongue lateralization. Ask the child to lift his tongue tip to his alveolar ridge.

Cheeks   Observe the tone of the cheeks at rest.

Palate   Determine if the child has a reported cleft of the hard palate. This might be a unilateral cleft, a bilateral cleft, or a sub-mucous cleft. A unilateral or bilateral cleft of the hard palate is almost certain to cause swallowing difficulties. (See Chapter 2.) Clefts of the soft palate may also cause feeding difficulties as the child may have difficulty obtaining velo-pharyngeal closure or closure of the palate against the base of the tongue for good oral pressure for sucking. If a child has had a prolonged oro-tracheal intubation, the tube may

Chapter 3: Clinical Evaluation of Infants and Children, *continued*

have caused a groove to form in the middle of the hard palate and alveolar ridge. This can interfere with sucking, or with older children, food may get stuck there.

Gums/Teeth   Some medications (e.g., seizure medications) can cause swelling in the gums. If the mouth is sore, the child is less likely to want to eat.

Note any significant decay in the teeth. If the child grinds his teeth, note if they are ground down to gum level. This may cause oral pain and decreased efficiency with masticated foods.

Respiration   Remove the child's shirt and observe if the child appears to be breathing adequately, showing some shallow breathing, showing extreme movement of the belly for belly breathing, showing reverse breathing (thoracic musculature appears to be breathing in while abdominal muscles are breathing out), or showing thoracic breathing in which the upper chest area moves excessively during breathing.

Hypersensitivity   Note the child's reaction to being touched on the face or in the mouth. Hypersensitivity may interfere with adequate feeding.

Nutritive Feeding Evaluation

Normal Reflexes   **rooting:** Note whether the child exhibits a rooting reflex when stimulated at the right, left, or at midline of lips. An absent or diminished reflex may indicate poor tactile sensation or integration of tactile stimuli (Wolf and Glass, 1992). If the child exhibits excessive rooting, he may have hypersensitivity or a lack of inhibition. Rooting should disappear between 3-6 months.

suckle-swallow: Touch your finger or the nipple lightly to the child's lips or tongue to see if suckling begins. If so, the finger or nipple will be drawn into the mouth and active suckling will be observed. If you get no response initially, evaluate again. The child may not have been alert enough or may not have been hungry. If a reduced suckling reflex or absent suckling reflex is consistently found, it usually indicates a neurological disorder (Wolf and Glass, 1992). Suckling should disappear between 6-12 months.

Chapter 3: Clinical Evaluation of Infants and Children, continued

Abnormal Reflexes Do not specifically elicit abnormal reflexes. Observe for the occurrence of any of these during feeding.

tonic bite: strong closure of the jaw when teeth or gums are stimulated; may be difficult for the child to release the bite

jaw thrust: strong downward extension of the lower jaw; jaw may appear to be stuck open

tongue retraction: strong pulling back of the tongue into the hypopharynx; the tip of the tongue may be held against the hard palate

tongue thrust: forceful protrusion of the tongue from the mouth

overactive gag: gag reflex stimulated in front of mouth

Feeding Position If the child utilizes a specialized seating device, describe it here. In particular, note whether the device provides lateral head support and trunk support, and whether it is at 90° or reclined slightly.

Note if the child is able to sit unsupported (this includes sitting in a regular high chair).

Bottle/Breast

Suck/Swallow/Breathe Pattern In young infants, the typical pattern is one suck, one swallow, and one pause for breathing. That is, the child sucks once to draw fluid into the mouth, stops breathing to swallow the fluid, and then breathes. In older infants, two or three sucks may occur per swallow.

Suckle/suck Between 6-9 months of age, the child should switch from an immature suckle pattern to a more mature suck. Note which is observed.

Burst cycles With nutritive sucking, a child usually shows an initial continuous sucking burst for at least the first 30 seconds, and sometimes as much as 60-80 seconds. That means that during the first minute, the child is showing a suck/swallow/breathe pattern continuing for up to 60-80 seconds before pausing to rest. As the child becomes satiated, the child then has fewer sucks in each burst and

Chapter 3: Clinical Evaluation of Infants and Children, *continued*

longer pauses (Mathew et al., 1985 and Shivpuri et al., 1983). By the end of a feeding, the child may be only showing two to three sucks in a burst.

Fluid expression   This is a subjective judgment. With bottle feeding, bubbles should be observed with each swallow. You have to judge whether the child is getting enough with each suck. A problem in this area may be indicated by a child who sucks three or four times before swallowing. This probably means that the infant is having to work too hard to express any of the fluid.

Anterior loss   Some loss around a nipple is normal for an infant. Mark if there is excessive loss.

Endurance   Endurance is related to the amount of liquid consumed and the length of time it takes a child to consume the liquid. Does the child stay alert throughout feeding without appearing fatigued? Each feeding should take no longer than 20 minutes.

Does the child consume an adequate amount before becoming fatigued? By the time infants are 3 months of age, they should be taking 7-8 ounces at each feeding.

Amount consumed
- 5 months: 9-10 ounces during each of 4-6 feedings a day
- 7 months: 11 or more ounces (food/liquid) during each of 4-6 feedings a day

Spoon

Removes food during spoon feeding   Beginning at 3 months, the child should use a suckling pattern as food touches the lips. By 9 months, the child should use more of a sucking pattern.

Waits quietly for the spoon   At 6-7 months, a child should wait quietly when he sees a spoon approaching. It is abnormal for the jaw to thrust forcefully open.

Lips assist in food removal   By 8 months, the child's upper lip should be touching the spoon and helping to remove food from the spoon. It is abnormal to have lip retraction with an inability to bring the lip down.

The Source for Pediatric Dysphagia

Chapter 3: Clinical Evaluation of Infants and Children, *continued*

Moves food posteriorly	At 4 months, some food is pushed out of the mouth as the child is using a suckle pattern. By 9 months, an up-and-down sucking pattern should be used with intermittent use of a protrusion/retraction pattern. At 12 months, some foods may be swallowed with the tongue tip elevated at times. By 18 months, the protrusion/retraction movement should be gone.
It is abnormal to have strong forward thrusting of the tongue or the tongue bunched and retracted at any age.
Cleans lower lip with top teeth	At 15 months, a child is able to do this.
Licks lips clean	At 24 months, a child should be able to do this.
Amount consumed	Does the child consume an adequate amount? Children 4-6 months of age should take one small serving of cereal a day. (A serving equals 2-3 tablespoons.) By 6-8 months, the child should take 2 servings of cereal, 1 fruit, and 2 vegetables. At 8-12 months, the child should take 2-3 servings of cereal, 2 fruits, 2-3 vegetables, and 2 meats.

Cup

Moves liquid with suckle/suck	A suckling pattern, or some mixture of suckling/sucking is used by 6-8 months. By 12 months, a true sucking pattern should be observed.
Extension/ retraction pattern of tongue	Extension and retraction should be seen by 6-8 months, but should disappear by about 12 months. It is abnormal to have a strong tongue thrust forward pattern or the tongue bunched and retracted in the mouth.
Anterior loss	It is normal for children to lose liquids anteriorly to some degree up until about 12 months of age.
Jaw opening graded/thrust	At 6-8 months of age, the child may still be opening his mouth very wide when a cup approaches. This should happen rarely by the time the child is 12 months of age. Strong forward jaw thrust is abnormal.
Stabilizes cup	At 12 months, the child may place his tongue slightly beneath the cup to help stabilize it. By 18 months, the child may bite down on the edge of the cup to stabilize it.

Chapter 3: Clinical Evaluation of Infants and Children, *continued*

Upper lip closes on edge of cup — At 18 months, the upper lip will close on the edge of the cup to provide a better seal for drinking. Lip retraction is abnormal.

Up-down sucking motion — By 24 months, a very coordinated up-and-down sucking pattern with the cup between the lips emerges.

Bite/Chew

Phasic bite pattern — At 5 months of age, a primitive phasic bite and release pattern is used.

Sustained bite pattern — At 10-12 months of age, the child may be able to use a controlled bite on a soft cookie. A controlled bite on a harder substance (e.g., a hard cookie or a pretzel) does not emerge until 13-15 months of age.

Moves food from tongue to chewing surface — By 7-9 months, the infant is seen to move food side to center or center to side using his tongue.

Diagonal/rotary chew — At 7-9 months, a diagonal/rotary chewing pattern may be emerging.

Moves food from one side to another — Between 19 and 24 months, the child may transfer food across one side through midline to the other side. The food usually pauses at midline.

Moves food posteriorly — This should be a fairly coordinated movement without much anterior loss. By at least 16-18 months, strong tongue thrusting or tongue bunching is abnormal.

Lips active during chewing — At 7-9 months, the child's lips appear to be active during chewing. The upper lip comes down and forward and both lips are drawn slightly inward.

Response to Feeding

Note the following responses to feeding: alert throughout, lethargic throughout, or irritable. Does the child demonstrate changes in respiratory function? Vomiting? Change in tone or other signs of distress?

Control of Oral Secretions

Sheppard (1995) suggests placing the child in a reclining position. This will prevent any anterior loss of secretions and will allow you to assess whether the child can initiate a swallow without the confounding factor of labial loss and ability to transport the saliva posteriorly in the oral cavity. If secretions are seen to be pooling in the posterior oral cavity, this may indicate a problem with initiating swallow. If the child sounds very wet and gurgly with secretions suspected to be pooling in the hypopharynx, there may be some pharyngeal phase disorder. Position the child upright and determine if there is any drooling which may show problems with other parts of the oral cavity. By 6 months, a child should drool only rarely in supine, prone, or sitting position. She may drool if she is babbling, using her hands, or manipulating objects. Keep in mind that children often drool when teething. By 9 months, the drooling should be occurring basically during teething, but not before or after.

Pharyngeal Symptoms

Note any pharyngeal symptoms. As in the adult population, children can also be silent aspirators. Arvedson et al. (1992) reviewed videofluoroscopic evaluations of 186 children. Aspiration was found in 48 of the children. The aspiration was silent in 45 of the 48.

Response to Compensations

If an infant is having difficulty during the assessment, you want to try some techniques to see if you can improve the child's performance. As in most assessments performed by SLPs, there is a component of stimulability testing which occurs. A more detailed description of these techniques is provided in Chapter 5 and Chapter 6. A short description is given here. On any compensation that you attempt, note the infant's response.

Support to lips	If the child is having excessive anterior loss, provide a little support at the corners of the lips to help the child get better closure.
External jaw support	Excessive anterior loss may also be caused by reduced jaw control. Place a finger lightly under the child's chin to provide some support.
External cheek support	Sometimes the child can't get good suction because of decreased tone in the cheeks. Using your thumb and middle finger on the hand which is holding the bottle, provide some support to the cheeks to help the child achieve some stability in his suck.
Change in posture	You might try a more flexed pattern with shoulders pulled forward and chin tucked to provide a little better airway protection. You might also try sidelying for the child with poor head control.
External pacing	External pacing may be accomplished by pulling the nipple away or tipping the bottle so there is no fluid in the nipple.

Chapter 3: Clinical Evaluation of Infants and Children, *continued*

	This technique is helpful for infants who seem to have a hard time organizing their suck/swallow/breathe pattern.
Calming/ organizing/ alerting	A variety of calming/organizing/alerting techniques are described in detail in Chapter 6. If a child is not in an appropriate state during the feeding, stop, use these techniques, and then try to continue the assessment. Older children may also benefit from techniques to create a conducive environment. (See Chapter 5, pages 129-130.)
Establish non-nutritive suck	If an infant is having difficulty coordinating suck/swallow/breathe when you present the bottle, stop and return to a non-nutritive suck on a pacifier or finger. This may help the child organize the suck/swallow/breathe pattern. You can then return to the assessment with nutritive sucking. Frequent breaks for burping may be needed and may even facilitate endurance. Use the burping break to introduce non-nutritive sucking to help the infant organize (Comrie and Helm, 1997).
Oral stimulation	For the child who fails to latch on (i.e., achieve tight closure with lips and tongue), providing some oral stimulation may increase the child's readiness for feeding. Oral stimulation can also help the child achieve better lip closure for spoon usage and cup drinking.
Negative resistance	Comrie and Helm (1997) describe a technique to use with infants who use a biting pattern rather than a sucking pattern or for infants who have an inefficient and rapid sucking pattern. Provide timed negative resistance during the infant's attempts to suck. As the infant pulls in the nipple slightly during sucking, gently tug on the nipple to create a stronger suck. If the technique is successful, longer and larger streams of bubbles should be observed. Never pull the nipple so hard that it comes out of the child's mouth or breaks the suction seal. This negative resistance may also facilitate organization and conserve energy. Comrie and Helm advise using this with firm jaw support.
Change in nipple	Avoid changing nipples numerous times during an assessment as this will only confuse the child. If one nipple seems very inappropriate (see Chapter 11), stop and give the infant a rest and then continue with a different type of nipple. Remember that the flow rate of the nipple can change breathing (Shivpuri et al. 1983). Mathew (1991) noted a decrease in the amount of breathing done in one minute with preemies using a high-flow nipple (preemie nipples are high-flow nipples). Mathew indicated that this may suggest that high-flow nipples yield a greater ventilatory compromise.

The Source for Pediatric Dysphagia

Chapter 3: Clinical Evaluation of Infants and Children, *continued*

Thicken liquids	Slightly thickening the liquids helps children who have poor motor control. It also helps infants with significant gastroesophageal reflux and projectile vomiting. Thickened liquids do not flow out of a cup as fast and therefore do not startle a child who is just learning cup drinking.
Change in utensils	Note any change in utensil and the child response. (See Chapter 11.)

Recommendations

Position the Child	Provide recommendations about the best way to position the child during feeding.
Use bottle/ nipple/pacifier/ cup/spoon	Describe the kind of nipple and pacifier you found to be most successful with the child. Most often you want to use the same shape pacifier nipple as you do on the bottle. List any other utensils found to be beneficial such as plate guards, weighted handle spoons, etc.
Types of food/ liquid	Identify the types of food the child was able to eat and drink (i.e., smooth, semi-chunky, mildly thick).
Frequency of feeding/ schedule	Considerations here include how quickly the child fatigues. If the child wears out and cannot finish the feeding, more frequent, shorter feedings may be indicated. Consult with the child's pediatrician or neonatologist and nursing staff to help determine the appropriate feeding schedule. Some children are allowed to eat throughout the day and do not have established meal patterns.
Environment	Note the environment which seemed the most appropriate. The child may need a calm environment without much background noise or movement in order to maintain an organized state. The child may also respond to rocking or to the use of music. For some children, rocking or music tends to decrease their level of alertness.
Stress signals	Note any stress signals the child exhibits which you recorded under *Response to Feeding*. Caregivers are not always aware that these kinds of movements indicate stress. Indicate how the feeder should respond to the stress signals.
Pacing	Note if the child seemed to need breaks.
Further Evaluation	Note if the child needs further diagnostic evaluations or consultations.

Chapter 3: Clinical Evaluation of Infants and Children, continued

Example Pediatric Feeding Evaluation (4 months and older)

Name: _Doris_ Patient #: _____ Date of Eval: _12-30-98_

DOB: _11-18-97_ Age: _13 months_ MD: _C. T. Mandu_

Medical History: _drug exposure prenatally - not addicted; delayed development of motor skills_

Feeding Patterns: _takes only bottles and smooth baby foods; takes bottle 7-8x day whenever she wants one_
Feeding Concerns Reported: _gags and "chokes" w/solids_

Structure/Function

Contractures
☐ yes ☐ no

Trunk
☐ tone
☐ lateral trunk flexion
☐ trunk rotation
☐ other: _____

Head Control
☐ midline
☐ other: _____

Jaw
☐ asymmetrical at rest
☐ thrust/asymmetry on opening
☐ cannot maintain closure

Lips
☐ asymmetry at rest
☐ cannot spread
☐ cannot pucker

Tongue
☐ asymmetrical at rest
☐ frenum restricts protrusion
☐ cannot protrude
☐ cannot elevate tip

Cheeks
☐ abnormal tone at rest

Palate
☐ cleft hard palate (uni/bi/sub)
☐ cleft soft palate

Gums/Teeth
☐ swollen/cracked
☐ decay
☐ ground

Respiration
☐ shallow breathing
☐ belly breathing
☐ reverse breathing
☐ thoracic breathing

Hypersensitivity
☑ face
☑ mouth

The Source for Pediatric Dysphagia

Chapter 3: Clinical Evaluation of Infants and Children, continued

Example Pediatric Feeding Evaluation (4 months and older), continued

Name: _Doris_

Nutritive Feeding Evaluation

Normal reflexes
☐ rooting (R/L/mid)
☐ suckle-swallow

Abnormal Reflexes
☐ tonic bite
☐ jaw thrust
☐ tongue retraction
☐ tongue thrust
☐ overactive gag

Feeding Position
____ supine with head elevated
____ prone
____ sidelying
____ reclined/elevated
✔ seating device at _90%_
____ sitting unsupported

(Bottle)/Breast (Circle one.)
Suck/Swallow/Breathe Pattern
_2-3_ # sucks to swallow
____ Suckle ✔ Suck
Burst cycles
initial burst: ____ 30 sec. ____ 45 sec. ✔ 60 sec.
____ follows normal pattern of steady decline
____ declines much too quickly
Fluid expression
✔ good ____ fair ____ poor
Anterior loss
____ normal ✔ excessive
Endurance
✔ adequate ____ decreased
Amount consumed
_6 oz._ in _10_ minutes

Spoon ____ CNA
Removes food with
✔ suckle ____ suck
Waits quietly for spoon
✔ yes ____ no
____ jaw thrust
Lips assist in food removal
✔ yes ____ no
Lips retracted ____ yes ____ no
Moves food posteriorly well
✔ yes ____ no
____ tongue thrust
____ tongue retracted
Cleans lower lip with top teeth
✔ yes ____ no
Licks lips clean
✔ yes ____ no
Amount consumed
1 jar in _10_ minutes

Response to Feeding
alert throughout ✔
lethargic _____
irritable ✔ _w/solids_
changes in respiratory function _____
vomiting _____
increased hypertonicity _____
increased hypotonicity _____
other signs of distress _gagging_

Cup ____ CNA
Moves liquid with
____ suckle ____ suck ✔ unable to use cup
Extension/retraction pattern of tongue
✔ yes ____ no
____ tongue thrust
____ tongue retracted
Anterior loss
____ normal ✔ excessive
Jaw opening graded ____ yes ✔ no
Jaw thrust ✔ yes ____ no
Stabilizes cup by
____ tongue under cup
✔ biting cup
Upper lip closes on edge of cup
____ yes ____ no
✔ lip retraction
Up-down sucking motion ____ yes ✔ no

Bite/Chew ____ CNA
Phasic bite pattern ____ yes ____ no ✔ CNA
Sustained bite pattern ____ yes ____ no ✔ CNA
Moves food from tongue to chewing surface
____ yes ✔ no
Diagonal/rotary chew ____ yes ✔ no
Moves food from one side to another
____ yes ✔ no
Moves food posteriorly
____ yes ✔ no
____ tongue thrust
____ tongue retracted
Lips active during chewing
✔ yes ____ no
Lips retracted ____ yes ____ no

Control of Oral Secretions
____ drooling
____ pooling in mouth/pharynx

Comments
_____
_____
_____
_____

The Source for Pediatric Dysphagia

Chapter 3: Clinical Evaluation of Infants and Children, *continued*

Example Pediatric Feeding Evaluation (4 months and older), *continued*

Name: _Doris_

Pharyngeal Symptoms

☐ congestion ☑ coughing/gagging ☐ multiple swallows ☐ wet vocal sounds
☐ wet breath sounds ✔ solids ___ liquids ☐ changes in breathing

Response to Compensations

Support to lips	
External jaw support	doesn't want face touched
External cheek support	
Change in posture (describe)	
External pacing	
pull nipple away	
bottle tipping	
Calming/organizing/alerting	
Establish non-nutritive suck	
Provide oral stimulation	
lip tap	
lingual stroke/tap	
Negative resistance	
Change in nipple (describe)	
Thicken liquids	for cup drinking - handled a little better
Change in utensils (describe)	
Other (describe)	

Recommendations

Position the child to feed: _in high chair_ Bottle: _regular_
Nipple: _regular_ Pacifier: _wean_ Cup: _cut-out_
Spoon: _small bowl_ Type(s) of food: _smooth_ Type(s) of liquid: _mildly thick from cup_
Frequency of feeding/schedule: _3x day plus snacks_ Environment: _reduce distractions_
Watch for these stress signals: _gagging, coughing_
Respond to stress signals by: _pending MBS_
Pacing: _n/a_ Other: _desensitize trunk, face, oral cavity; eat before getting bottle_
Further evaluation: _MBS to assess aspiration_

_____ _____ _____ _____
SLP   Date   Time   Procedure

Chapter 3: Clinical Evaluation of Infants and Children, continued

Pediatric Feeding Evaluation (4 months and older)

Name: _____ Patient #: _____ Date of Eval: _____

DOB: _____ Age: _____ MD: _____

Medical History: _____
_____
_____

Feeding Patterns: _____
Feeding Concerns Reported: _____

Structure/Function

Contractures
- ☐ yes ☐ no

Trunk
- ☐ tone
- ☐ lateral trunk flexion
- ☐ trunk rotation
- ☐ other: _____

Head Control
- ☐ midline
- ☐ other: _____

Jaw
- ☐ asymmetrical at rest
- ☐ thrust/asymmetry on opening
- ☐ cannot maintain closure

Lips
- ☐ asymmetry at rest
- ☐ cannot spread
- ☐ cannot pucker

Tongue
- ☐ asymmetrical at rest
- ☐ frenum restricts protrusion
- ☐ cannot protrude
- ☐ cannot elevate tip

Cheeks
- ☐ abnormal tone at rest

Palate
- ☐ cleft hard palate (uni/bi/sub)
- ☐ cleft soft palate

Gums/Teeth
- ☐ swollen/cracked
- ☐ decay
- ☐ ground

Respiration
- ☐ shallow breathing
- ☐ belly breathing
- ☐ reverse breathing
- ☐ thoracic breathing

Hypersensitivity
- ☐ face
- ☐ mouth

The Source for Pediatric Dysphagia

Chapter 3: Clinical Evaluation of Infants and Children, continued

Pediatric Feeding Evaluation (4 months and older), continued

Name: _____

Nutritive Feeding Evaluation

Normal reflexes
☐ rooting (R/L/mid)
☐ suckle-swallow

Abnormal Reflexes
☐ tonic bite
☐ jaw thrust
☐ tongue retraction
☐ tongue thrust
☐ overactive gag

Feeding Position
____ supine with head elevated
____ prone
____ sidelying
____ reclined/elevated
____ seating device at _____
____ sitting unsupported

Bottle/Breast (Circle one.)
Suck/Swallow/Breathe Pattern
____ # sucks to swallow
____ Suckle   ____ Suck
Burst cycles
initial burst: ____ 30 sec.   ____ 45 sec.   ____ 60 sec.
____ follows normal pattern of steady decline
____ declines much too quickly
Fluid expression
____ good   ____ fair   ____ poor
Anterior loss
____ normal   ____ excessive
Endurance
____ adequate   ____ decreased
Amount consumed
____ in ____ minutes

Spoon ____ CNA
Removes food with
____ suckle   ____ suck
Waits quietly for spoon
____ yes   ____ no
____ jaw thrust
Lips assist in food removal
____ yes   ____ no
Lips retracted   ____ yes   ____ no
Moves food posteriorly well
____ yes   ____ no
____ tongue thrust
____ tongue retracted
Cleans lower lip with top teeth
____ yes   ____ no
Licks lips clean
____ yes   ____ no
Amount consumed
____ in ____ minutes

Cup ____ CNA
Moves liquid with
____ suckle   ____ suck   ____ unable to use cup
Extension/retraction pattern of tongue
____ yes   ____ no
____ tongue thrust
____ tongue retracted
Anterior loss
____ normal   ____ excessive
Jaw opening graded ____ yes ____ no
Jaw thrust ____ yes ____ no
Stabilizes cup by
____ tongue under cup
____ biting cup
Upper lip closes on edge of cup
____ yes   ____ no
____ lip retraction
Up-down sucking motion ____ yes ____ no

Bite/Chew ____ CNA
Phasic bite pattern ____ yes ____ no ____ CNA
Sustained bite pattern ____ yes ____ no ____ CNA
Moves food from tongue to chewing surface
____ yes   ____ no
Diagonal/rotary chew ____ yes ____ no
Moves food from one side to another
____ yes   ____ no
Moves food posteriorly
____ yes   ____ no
____ tongue thrust
____ tongue retracted
Lips active during chewing
____ yes   ____ no
Lips retracted ____ yes ____ no

Response to Feeding
alert throughout _____
lethargic _____
irritable _____
changes in respiratory function _____
vomiting _____
increased hypertonicity _____
increased hypotonicity _____
other signs of distress _____

Control of Oral Secretions
____ drooling
____ pooling in mouth/pharynx

Comments
_____
_____
_____
_____

The Source for Pediatric Dysphagia

Chapter 3: Clinical Evaluation of Infants and Children, continued

Pediatric Feeding Evaluation (4 months and older), continued

Name: _____

Pharyngeal Symptoms

☐ congestion ☐ coughing/gagging ☐ multiple swallows ☐ wet vocal sounds
☐ wet breath sounds ___ solids ___ liquids ☐ changes in breathing

Response to Compensations

Support to lips	
External jaw support	
External cheek support	
Change in posture (describe)	
External pacing	
pull nipple away	
bottle tipping	
Calming/organizing/alerting	
Establish non-nutritive suck	
Provide oral stimulation	
lip tap	
lingual stroke/tap	
Negative resistance	
Change in nipple (describe)	
Thicken liquids	
Change in utensils (describe)	
Other (describe)	

Recommendations

Position the child to feed: _____ Bottle: _____
Nipple: _____ Pacifier: _____ Cup: _____
Spoon: _____ Type(s) of food: _____ Type(s) of liquid: _____
Frequency of feeding/schedule: _____ Environment: _____
Watch for these stress signals: _____
Respond to stress signals by: _____
Pacing: _____ Other: _____
Further evaluation: _____

_____ _____ _____ _____
SLP   Date   Time   Procedure

The Source for Pediatric Dysphagia

Chapter 3: Clinical Evaluation of Infants and Children, continued

Example Case History/Interview Form for Children with Feeding Problems (4 months and older)

Name: __Doris__

DOB: __11-18-97__   Age: __13 months__

Address: _____

Caregiver(s): __foster mother__

Home phone: _____   Work phone: _____

Primary care physician: __H. I. Persensitive__

Other physicians treating child: __has seen ENT__

Why is your child being seen for a feeding evaluation? __won't/can't drink from cup, won't eat solids - gags__

Medical History

Has your child had any surgeries? ____ yes   __✔__ no

If *yes*, please list with dates: _____

Has your child ever been hospitalized? ____ yes   __✔__ no

If *yes*, please list reason(s) and date(s): _____

Is your child on any medication? ____ yes   __✔__ no

If *yes*, please list: _____

Does your child have any allergies (food or otherwise)? ____ yes   __✔__ no

If *yes*, please list: _____

Birth History

Weight of your child at birth: __5 lbs., 1 oz.__

Was your child full-term? __✔__ yes   ____ no

If *no*, how many weeks gestation? _____

Were there any problems during pregnancy? __✔__ yes   ____ no

If *yes*, please describe: __Mom took drugs__

Were there any problems immediately after birth? ____ yes   __✔__ no

If *yes*, please describe: _____

Chapter 3: Clinical Evaluation of Infants and Children, continued

Example Case History (4 months and older), continued

Developmental History
Please indicate ages:

sitting unsuppported _8 1/2 months_   walking _not yet_

crawling _10 months_   self-dressing _not yet_

standing alone _12 months_   bladder and bowel control _not yet_

Feeding History

Was your child breast-fed? ____ yes   _✔_ no

If *yes*, how long? _____ Were there any problems with this (e.g., poor suck, slow to feed)? _____

When was your child first given a bottle? _birth_   Were there any problems with this (e.g., poor suck, slow to feed)? _we didn't get her until 7 weeks, took a long time to feed her_

When did your child start to eat solid foods? _tried at 6 months_

Were there any problems with this? _child gagged and choked_

When was your child weaned from bottle/breast? _still takes bottle_

When did the child start to feed him/herself? _not yet_

Does the child drink juice? _✔_ yes ____ no If *yes*, how much in a day? _8 oz._

Is the juice given (before), (during), or (after) a meal? (Please circle.)

Does your child exhibit any of the following behaviors:

____ crying	_✔_ spitting food out of his/her mouth	____ holding food in his/her mouth
_✔_ gagging		
____ vomiting	____ regurgitating food	____ getting down from the table during meal

How many times a day does your child eat? _3-4 times_

If your child does not feed him/herself, who feeds him/her? _I do_

Where does your child eat? _in kitchen with us_

How is your child positioned when eating (e.g., sitting in high chair, sitting on the floor)?
high chair or stroller

Who else is present for meals? _rest of family_

The Source for Pediatric Dysphagia

Chapter 3: Clinical Evaluation of Infants and Children, *continued*

Example Case History (4 months and older), *continued*

Does your child eat more/less,(same)/different foods when he/she is at daycare/ baby-sitter/(grandparents)/other? (Please circle and describe. gags with everybody

_____

_____ ✔ _____

Does your child receive supplemental (tube) feeding: _____ yes _____ no

If *yes*, amount _____   NG: _____

    rate _____   PEG: _____

                  PEJ: _____

Bolus (given via syringe several times a day): _____

Continuous (connected to pump): _____

What consistency of foods does your child eat?   How is liquid presented?

regular liquids ✔   ✔ bottle *regular*

thickened liquids _____   ✔ type of nipple *regular*

baby cereal _____   _____ breast

Stage 1 baby foods (smooth) ✔   _____ cup

Stage 2 baby foods (semi-chunky) _____   _____ spout

Stage 3 baby foods (chunky) _____   _____ lid with no spout

mashed table food _____   _____ cut-out cup

regular table food _____

Approximately how much liquid does your child drink at each meal? *1 bottle*

Approximately how much food does your child eat at each meal? *2 1/2 jars of food*

How long does each meal take? *20-30 minutes*

What do you do when your child does not eat appropriately? *stop giving her the food with lumps*

_____

What are some of your child's favorite foods? *smooth banana yogurt, baby green beans, baby fruits*

_____

If different from favorite foods, what are some easy foods for your child to eat? _____

   anything that doesn't have pieces in it

The Source for Pediatric Dysphagia

Chapter 3: Clinical Evaluation of Infants and Children, *continued*

Example Case History (4 months and older), *continued*

Which foods will your child not eat? _yogurt with fruit, baby cereal, cookies, pretzels_

If different from foods that your child will not eat, what are some difficult foods for your child to eat? _____

List some good things that your child does at meal times (e.g., sits at the table, eats certain foods). _stays in high chair_

List some things that you think your child should be doing at meal times that he/she does not do (e.g., eating different kinds of foods). _eating Stage 2 baby foods and some solids_

List some things that you think your child should not be doing at meals (e.g., having a tantrum, throwing food). _gagging_

What have you tried to do to help your child with his/her feeding problem?
crushed up the crackers and cookies

Please describe any other feeding problem(s) that your child is experiencing.

Person completing form: _____

Date: _____

Chapter 3: Clinical Evaluation of Infants and Children, continued

Case History/Interview Form for Children with Feeding Problems (4 months and older)

Name: _____

DOB: _____ Age: _____

Address: _____

Caregiver(s): _____

Home phone: _____ Work phone: _____

Primary care physician: _____

Other physicians treating child: _____

Why is your child being seen for a feeding evaluation? _____

_____

Medical History

Has your child had any surgeries? _____ yes _____ no

If *yes*, please list with dates: _____

_____

Has your child ever been hospitalized? _____ yes _____ no

If *yes*, please list reason(s) and date(s): _____

_____

Is your child on any medication? _____ yes _____ no

If *yes*, please list: _____

Does your child have any allergies (food or otherwise)? _____ yes _____ no

If *yes*, please list: _____

Birth History

Weight of your child at birth _____

Was your child full-term? _____ yes _____ no

If *no*, how many weeks gestation? _____

Were there any problems during pregnancy? _____ yes _____ no

If *yes*, please describe: _____

Were there any problems immediately after birth? _____ yes _____ no

If *yes*, please describe: _____

The Source for Pediatric Dysphagia

Chapter 3: Clinical Evaluation of Infants and Children, *continued*

Case History (4 months and older), *continued*

Developmental History
Please indicate ages:

sitting unsuppported _____   walking _____

crawling _____   self-dressing _____

standing alone _____   bladder and bowel control _____

Feeding History

Was your child breast-fed? _____ yes   _____ no

If *yes*, how long? _____ Were there any problems with this (e.g., poor suck, slow to feed)? _____

When was your child first given a bottle? _____ Were there any problems with this (e.g., poor suck, slow to feed)? _____

When did your child start to eat solid foods? _____

Were there any problems with this? _____

When was your child weaned from bottle/breast? _____

When did the child start to feed him/herself? _____

Does the child drink juice? _____ yes   _____ no If *yes*, how much in a day? _____

Is the juice given before, during, or after a meal? (Please circle.)

Does your child exhibit any of the following behaviors:

_____ crying   _____ spitting food out of his/her mouth   _____ holding food in his/her mouth

_____ gagging

_____ vomiting   _____ regurgitating food   _____ getting down from the table during meal

How many times a day does your child eat? _____

If your child does not feed him/herself, who feeds him/her? _____

Where does your child eat? _____

How is your child positioned when eating (e.g., sitting in high chair, sitting on the floor)? _____

Who else is present for meals? _____

The Source for Pediatric Dysphagia

Chapter 3: Clinical Evaluation of Infants and Children, continued

Case History (4 months and older), continued

Does your child eat more/less, same/different foods when he/she is at daycare/ baby-sitter/grandparents/other? (Please circle and describe.) _____

_____

Does your child receive supplemental (tube) feeding: ____ yes   ____ no

If *yes*, amount _____   NG: _____

    rate _____   PEG: _____

                       PEJ: _____

Bolus (given via syringe several times a day): _____

Continuous (connected to pump): _____

What consistency of foods does your child eat?   How is liquid presented?

regular liquids ____   ____ bottle _____

thickened liquids ____   ____ type of nipple _____

baby cereal ____   ____ breast

Stage 1 baby foods (smooth) ____   ____ cup

Stage 2 baby foods (semi-chunky) ____   ____ spout

Stage 3 baby foods (chunky) ____   ____ lid with no spout

mashed table food ____   ____ cut-out cup

regular table food ____

Approximately how much liquid does your child drink at each meal? _____

Approximately how much food does your child eat at each meal? _____

How long does each meal take? _____

What do you do when your child does not eat appropriately? _____

_____

What are some of your child's favorite foods? _____

_____

If different from favorite foods, what are some easy foods for your child to eat? _____

_____

The Source for Pediatric Dysphagia

Chapter 3: Clinical Evaluation of Infants and Children, *continued*

Case History (4 months and older), *continued*

Which foods will your child not eat? _____

_____

If different from foods that your child will not eat, what are some difficult foods for your child to eat? _____

_____

List some good things that your child does at meal times (e.g., sits at the table, eats certain foods). _____

_____

List some things that you think your child should be doing at meal times that he/she does not do (e.g., eating different kinds of foods). _____

_____

List some things that you think your child should not be doing at meals (e.g., having a tantrum, throwing food). _____

_____

What have you tried to do to help your child with his/her feeding problem?

_____

_____

Please describe any other feeding problem(s) that your child is experiencing.

_____

_____

Person completing form: _____

Date: _____

Chapter 3: Clinical Evaluation of Infants and Children, continued

Appendix 3-A

Interpretation of Feeding History

Cluster of Symptoms: *Suggests need for:*

- parent description of swallowing problem
- gulping sounds
- noisy breathing only with feeding
- takes pacifier well, won't take bottle
- excessive drooling, need for oral suctioning
- history of respiratory illness: pneumonia, asthma, etc.

Careful assessment of swallow

- sleepy baby
- poor cues re: when to feed
- difficulty with feeding transitions
- agitated, cries a lot, sleeps poorly
- difficulty initiating sucking
- poor rhythm

Careful assessment of state/behavior

- parent describes sucking problem
- history of frequent changes of nipple
- history of enlarging nipple hole
- difficulty initiating sucking

Careful assessment of oral-motor control

- frequent spitting up, vomiting
- agitated, excessive crying
- sleeps poorly
- draws knees to chest with crying

Consider presence of GERD

- sleepy baby
- falls asleep prior to taking full feed
- sweating
- many colds
- chronic nasal congestion
- sucking becomes disorganized in middle of feeding
- slow sucking rhythm
- feeding lasts longer than 30 minutes

Careful assessment of endurance

- likes spoon better than sucking
- chronic nasal congestion
- uneven sucking rhythm
- baby forgets to breathe
- coughing, choking

Careful assessment of coordination of sucking, swallowing, and breathing

- excessive gagging
- very particular about nipple shape
- problems with transitions, especially to spoon
- history of tube feeding

Careful assessment of tactile responses

- color change has been noted
- baby forgets to breathe
- medical history of apnea and/or bradycardia with feed
- sweating

Assessment of physiologic parameters

- baby is fed too often
- baby not fed frequently enough
- baby not given adequate amount of formula, though parent perceives it as adequate
- inappropriate feeding position

Careful assessment of parent knowledge regarding infant feeding needs

From *Feeding and Swallowing Disorders in Infancy: Assessment and Management.* Copyright © 1992 by Therapy Skill Builders, a division of The Psychological Corporation. Reproduced by permission. All rights reserved.

Chapter 3: Clinical Evaluation of Infants and Children, continued

References

Alexander, R. "Oral-Motor and Feeding/Swallowing Function in the Young Child: Assessment and Intervention Strategies." Double Seminar presented at the Illinois Speech-Language-Hearing Association, 1998.

Apgar, V. "The Newborn (Apgar) Scoring System: Reflections and Advice." *Pediatric Clinics of North America*, Vol. 14, 1966, p. 645.

Arvedson, J.C. "Oral-Motor and Feeding Assessment." In Arvedson, J.C. and Brodsky, L. (eds.) *Pediatric Swallowing and Feeding: Assessment and Management*, San Diego: Singular Publishing Group, Inc., 1993, pp. 249-293.

Arvedson, J.C. et al. "Anatomy, Embryology, and Physiology." In Arvedson, J.C. and Brodsky, L. (eds.) *Pediatric Swallowing and Feeding: Assessment and Management*, San Diego: Singular Publishing Group, 1993, pp. 5-12.

Arvedson, J.C. et al. "Pediatric Dysphagia: 186 Videofluoro Swallow Studies." Paper presented at the American Speech-Language-Hearing Association Convention, San Antonio, Texas, 1992.

Boner, M.M. and Perlin, W.S. "Oral-Motor and Swallowing Skills in the Infant and Child: An Overview." In Cherney, L.R. (ed.) *Clinical Management of Dysphagia in Children and Adults*, Gaithersburg, MD: Aspen Publishers, 1994, pp. 29-49.

Brake, S. et al. "The First Nutritive Sucking Responses of Premature Newborns." *Infant Behavior and Development*, Vol. 9, 1988, pp. 1-9.

Brazelton, T.B. *Neonatal Behavioral Assessment Scale*, Philadelphia: J.D. Lippincott Company, 1984.

Bryan, D.W. and Pressman, H. "Comprehensive Team Evaluation." In Rosenthal, S. et al. (eds.) *Dysphagia and the Child with Developmental Disabilities: Medical, Clinical and Family Interventions*, San Diego: Singular Publishing Group, Inc., 1995, pp. 37-77.

Chow, M.P. et al. *Handbook of Pediatric Primary Care*, New York: John Wiley & Sons, 1984.

Comrie, J.D. and Helm, J.M. "Common Feeding Problems in the Intensive Care Nursery: Maturization, Organization, Evaluation, and Management Strategies." *Seminars in Speech and Language*, Vol. 18, No. 3, 1997, pp. 239-261.

Couriel, J.M. et al. "Assessment of Feeding Problems in Neurodevelopmental Handicap: A Team Approach." *Archives of Disease in Childhood*, Vol. 69, 1993, pp. 609-613.

Donner, M.W. "Editorial." *Dysphagia*, Vol. 1, 1986, pp. 1-2.

Finnie, N. *Handling the Young Cerebral Palsy Child at Home*, 7th ed, New York: E.P. Dutton, 1987, p. 122.

Klauss, M. and Fanaroff, A.A. *Care of the High Risk Neonate*, Philadelphia: W.B. Saunders, 1978.

Chapter 3: Clinical Evaluation of Infants and Children, continued

Krane, L.D. "Cardiopulmonary Management of the High Risk Neonate: Implications for Developmental Therapists." *Physical and Occupational Therapy in Pediatrics*, Vol. 6, 1986, pp. 255-281.

Kramer, S.F. and Eicher, P.M. "The Evaluation of Pediatric Feeding Abnormalities." *Dysphagia*, Vol. 3, 1993, pp. 215-224.

Lau, C. and Chanler, R.J. "Oral-Motor Function in the Neonate." *Neonatal Gastroenterology*, Vol. 23, No. 2, 1996, pp. 161-179.

Lefton-Grief, M.A. "Diagnosis and Management of Pediatric Feeding and Swallowing Disorders: Role of a SLP." In Tuchman, D. and Walter, R. (eds.) *Disorders of Feeding and Swallowing in Infants and Children*, San Diego: Singular Publishing Group, Inc., 1994, pp. 97-115.

Marx, K.H. "Growth of Sick, Premature Infants." In Cohen, S.A. (ed.) *The Underweight Infant, Child and Adolescent*, Norwalk, CT: Appleton-Century-Croft, 1986, pp. 56-65.

Mathison, B. et al. "Oral-Motor Dysfunction and Failure to Thrive Among Inner-city Infants." *Developmental Medicine and Child Neurology*, Vol. 231, 1989, pp. 293-302.

Mathew, O.P. "Breathing Patterns of Pre-term Infants During Bottle Feeding: Role of Milk Flow." *The Journal of Pediatrics*, Vol. 119, 1991, pp. 960-965.

Mathew, O.P. et al. "Breathing Pattern and Ventilation During Oral Feeding in Term Infants." *The Journal of Pediatrics*, Vol. 106, 1985, pp. 810-813.

Morris, S.E. "Developmental Implication for the Management of Feeding Problems in Neurologically Impaired Infants." *Seminars in Speech and Language*, Vol. 6, No. 4, 1985, pp. 293-315.

Morris, S.E. *The Normal Acquisition of Oral Feeding Skills: Implications for Assessment and Treatment*, Santa Barbara, CA: Therapeutic Media, Inc., 1981, pp. 99-102.

Morris, S.E. and Klein, M.D. *Pre-Feeding Skills: A Comprehensive Resource for Feeding Development*, San Antonio: Therapy Skill Builders, a division of The Psychological Corporation, 1987.

Nelson, C.A. and DeBeenabib, R.M. "Sensory Preparation of the Oral-Motor Area." In Langley, M.B. and Lombardino, L.J. (eds.) *Neurodevelopmental Strategies for Managing Communications Disorders in Children with Severe Motor Dysfunction*, Austin, TX: Pro-Ed, 1991, pp. 131-158.

Perlin, W.S. and Boner, M.M. "Clinical Assessment of Feeding and Swallowing in Infants and Children." In Cherney, L.R. (ed.) *Clinical Management of Dysphagia in Children and Adults*. Gaithersburg, MD: Aspen Publishers, 1994, pp. 93-133.

Rosen, C.L. et al. "Hypoxemia Associated with Feeding in the Pre-term and Full-term Neonate." *American Journal of Diseases in Children*, Vol. 138, 1984, pp. 623-628.

Selley, W.G. and Boxall, J. "A New Way to Treat Sucking and Swallowing Difficulties in Babies." *The Lancet*, Vol. 1, 1991, pp. 1182-1184.

Chapter 3: Clinical Evaluation of Infants and Children, continued

Sheppard, J.J. "Clinical Evaluation and Treatment." In Rosenthal, S. et al. (eds.) *Dysphagia and the Child with Developmental Disabilities: Medical, Clinical and Family Interventions.* San Diego: Singular Publishing Group, Inc., 1995, pp. 37-77.

Shivpuri, C.R. et al. "Decreased Ventilation in Pre-term Infants During Oral Feeding." *The Journal of Pediatrics,* Vol. 103, 1983, pp. 285-289.

Tuchman, D. and Walter, R. "Disorders of Deglutition." In Tuchman, D. and Walter, R. (eds.) *Disorders of Feeding and Swallowing in Infants and Children: Pathophysiology, Diagnosis and Treatment.* San Diego: Singular Publishing Group, Inc., 1994, pp. 53-77.

White-Traut, R.C. and Hutchens, C.M. "Modulating Infant State in Premature Infants." *Journal of Pediatric Nursing,* Vol. 2, 1987, pp. 96-101.

Wilson, J.M. *Oral-Motor Function and Dysfunction in Children,* Chapel Hill, NC: University of North Carolina, Division of Physical Therapy, 1978.

Wolf, L.F. and Glass, R.P. *Feeding and Swallowing Disorders in Infancy: Assessment and Management,* San Antonio: Therapy Skill Builders, a division of The Psychological Corporation, 1992.

Chapter 4: Instrumentation, Devices, and Diagnostic Procedures

As with the adult population, the results of a clinical evaluation of an infant or child sometimes indicate the need for further diagnostic evaluation. This further diagnostic work-up may be performed by the SLP (e.g., MBS study), or may require a referral to another medical specialist such as an otolaryngologist. This chapter describes the procedure for MBS and provides information about procedures performed by other medical specialists. This chapter also explains instrumentation and devices with which the SLP should be familiar when working with infants and children with dysphagia. These include monitors, feeding tubes, and other devices.

Modified Barium Swallow (MBS)

The MBS, or videofluoroscopic evaluation of swallowing, is both a diagnostic and a therapeutic procedure. If it were simply a diagnostic procedure, the study would be terminated as soon as aspiration was observed. The most important information obtained during an MBS comes after that point. This is when the SLP begins to try different compensations to determine if the child can eat or drink anything safely. The techniques might include changes in posture, texture, or presentation of food and liquid. The MBS allows assessment of the oral preparatory phase, oral (voluntary) phase, and the pharyngeal phase. It should also allow for screening of esophageal function.

MBS vs. Barium Swallow or Upper GI

A barium swallow assesses the esophagus and the stomach. An upper GI (UGI) assesses the stomach and the intestines. Because of the inter-relationship between disorders in the esophageal and pharyngeal phases, an MBS study should include at least a screening of the esophagus. For example, a referring complaint might be gagging behavior, vomiting, and inability to complete a meal. It would be impossible to determine from this symptomatology whether the disorder was limited to the pharyngeal phase or the esophageal phase. Very often it is a disorder in both, or an esophageal disorder which presents as pharyngeal symptoms. Therefore, it would be appropriate to assess the pharyngeal phase and screen the esophageal phase.

Goals of MBS

Logemann (1986) and Linden (1989) summarize the goals of an MBS:

- To define the nature and physiology of the impaired swallow

- To stress the system to try to recreate the presenting complaint

- To find compensations and adaptations that will help the child perform the best so a treatment plan can be established

Chapter 4: Instrumentation, Devices, and Diagnostic Procedures, continued

Before the Study

A complete history must be obtained from the medical record and from a caregiver interview before the study is completed. If you have already clinically evaluated this child, you probably have the complete history. If not, the case histories on pages 86-87 (infant) and 109-112 (pediatric) may be helpful to you when gathering information from the medical chart and through parent interview.

It is preferable that the child has a complete clinical evaluation before coming for the MBS study. This may have been completed by another SLP. If so, obtain complete results.

Try to schedule the MBS evaluation on a day and time that the child can exhibit optimum skills and fully participate. The child should be in good health. Some children are just not ready for an MBS study. If they are unable to stay alert long enough for eating, they are probably not ready for an MBS study.

Preparing the Child for the Study

In order to have the child remain as calm as possible, invite the caregiver into the fluoroscopy suite. If the child is old enough, it will be worth the investment of time to allow the child time to explore the videofluoroscopy table, VCR, monitor, etc., before the radiologist comes into the room to begin the study. Fully explain the procedure to the caregiver and any other observers. If the child is hospitalized, the child's nurse may want to observe the study as well. This is an excellent way to provide education to the nursing staff about the purpose of the MBS and about dysphagia in general. When the study is about to begin, changes in the lighting should be made gradually. Turning the lights off immediately is sure to frighten a child (Benson and Lefton-Grief, 1994).

What the Caregiver Should Bring

Ask the caregiver to bring the bottle, nipple, cup, spoon, etc. that the child usually uses to eat. Using these more familiar utensils will help the child feel at ease. Also ask the caregiver to bring things the child likes to eat in each of the texture categories you want to assess (e.g., If you want to check solids, ask the caregiver to bring a small sample of the kind of solid food the child eats.). You can mix barium paste or powder with any food. If the child has a particular preference about temperature of food, simulate that, too.

Preparation for the Study

It is not necessary for the child to have an empty stomach to perform an MBS, but an MBS is often done in combination with an upper GI series, and an empty stomach is needed for the upper GI series. The MBS study is done first so if any aspiration occurs, compensations can be made. This is immediately followed by the upper GI study.

While an empty stomach is not necessary for a child who is only having an MBS, it is helpful if the child is somewhat hungry. The child may be more willing to take the foods mixed with barium, which will taste strange to the child, if she is hungry. Therefore, you may want to make sure the child hasn't eaten for about two hours before coming in for the study. As suggested by Jolly, et al. (1995), holding an infant's feeding for over three hours may cause increased irritability and may interfere with the success of the study.

Medications

The child should take his medications, even if they are to be NPO for an upper GI. If the child is on an anti-reflux drug or esophageal motility drug, consult with the pediatrician to determine whether the child should take the medication before the MBS (Marquis and Pressman, 1995). If the goal of the esophageal screening portion of the study is to determine the degree of reflux, then perhaps it would be best not to have the child take the reflux medications. If the goal is to determine if the reflux and motility medications are helping to address the problem, then of course the child should take the medication.

Positioning the Child

Depending upon the age of the child and the child's ability to sit, a variety of options are available for positioning the child for the study. An infant or child under 60 pounds can be positioned in a Tumble Form® Chair that is placed on the footboard of the video fluoroscopy table. Many children's car seats may also serve the same purpose. Older children can be positioned in the Hausted® Chair. An infant can also be held by the caregiver. Be sure the caregiver wears a lead apron and is not pregnant at the time of the examination.

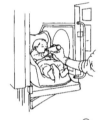
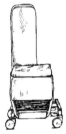

Tumble Form®

Hausted®

The infant can be held with her back against her parent's chest and the Radiology Technologist can present the food and liquid. A smaller child can also

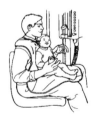
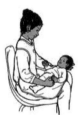

be held facing the parent and the parent can present the food or liquid. Older children who are able to sit independently may sit on the footboard. However, unless they are extremely cooperative, they are probably going to try to get up from the footboard.

On occasion, a child's specialized wheelchair will fit between the camera and the fluoroscopy table, but very often this does not allow for an A/P view because the chairs don't allow X-ray beams to penetrate.

It is important to try to simulate the position in which the child is fed most often to obtain information helpful in treatment planning. If you complete the study

Chapter 4: Instrumentation, Devices, and Diagnostic Procedures, continued

with the child at a 90° upright angle, and this is never how the child is fed, then you have not obtained the necessary information. If the presenting complaint is that the child's skills deteriorate toward the end of a meal, simulate the situation, but do not expose the child to greater amount of radiation. This can be done by making a video recording of the first several swallows of each texture. Then turn off the fluoroscopy and feed the child (it is not necessary to feed material with the barium in it) until the point at which the child begins to show difficulty. Then return to presenting barium-impregnated materials and begin recording again.

After examination in an upright position, place the infant in sidelying (on the right side) for further assessment of the esophageal phase. If the child has been particularly wiggly in upright, it may be necessary to view the child in sidelying for the pharyngeal phase as well.

Preparing the Barium Materials

Consistency	Comments
Liquid	Liquid barium may be presented by itself or mixed with the child's formula or fruit juice to mask the taste.
Thickened Liquid	The thin liquid mixture described above may be thickened with a commercial thickener or with some rice cereal. If the material is thickened too much, it will not pass through a nipple.
Pureed	Powdered barium or barium paste can be mixed with pureed baby food or pureed fruit. Choosing food that the child likes and that has a strong flavor will help mask the taste of the barium.
Pudding Thick	Commercial thickener or baby cereal can be used to thicken any liquid mixed with barium to the desired consistency.
Chewable Foods	Barium powder or paste can be mixed with any chewable foods (e.g., Stage 2 foods). Instead of spreading barium paste on a cookie, you can use cookies with barium powder baked into them. (See Appendix 4-A, page 126 for recipe.) The disadvantage to using barium smeared on a cookie is that the child will usually suck off and swallow the barium paste first, leaving you with a solid that cannot be visualized.

Radiation Dosage/Safety

Exposure to radiation is inevitable during an MBS, but it is important to keep radiation exposure to a minimum. Exposure to radiation only occurs when the fluoroscopy is on. The use of lead aprons to protect other body parts of the patients allows extra protection from scattered radiation outside the primary beam (Marquis and Pressman, 1995). Full assessment of the oral and pharyngeal phases of the swallow will require an average of five minutes of fluoroscopy time (Beck and Gayler, 1991). If the child is also to have an assessment of the esophagus, stomach, or intestines, the time will increase.

The individual who is presenting the material to the infant should wear lead gloves. Choose lead gloves that look like brown latex gloves and allow the flexibility needed to feed a child. The usual bulky, large lead gloves do not allow for adequate manipulation of the spoon or cup. Lead aprons and thyroid shields should also be available for anyone else in the fluoroscopy suite. The SLP and staff who repeatedly perform these studies should also wear film badges.

Order of Presentation

Thin liquids should be given in small amounts first, gradually increasing the amount. With children who are less than cooperative, you may not be able to go through the full range of materials you wish to present. This may force you to try uncontrolled amounts sooner than is typical. If the child is thought to be at extreme risk for aspiration of thin liquids, then it may be advisable to start with one of the thicker liquids. However, the disadvantage to this is that the valleculae and pyriform sinuses may become full and you will not be able to observe a thin liquid swallow as accurately.

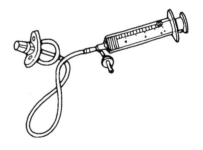

Marquis and Pressman (1995) describe a creative way to present liquid to an infant who refuses to take it once she tastes the barium. If the child will accept a nipple, a catheter is fed through a hole in the nipple and held in place with a clamp. The other end of the catheter is attached to a syringe. Small amounts of liquid can be introduced via the syringe. Often the child will then begin to initiate sucking. Even if the child will not suck, material can be dispensed through the syringe. Be very cautious and do not present too much liquid at once. In older children who refuse to take the material from a cup, a small catheter can be placed at the side of the tongue and liquid can be given slowly via syringe.

Careful Monitoring of Infant's Response

The response of the infant needs to be monitored very carefully. Premature infants in particular can decompensate very quickly. If the infant chokes or coughs a lot and becomes very upset, her oxygen saturation levels may decrease and she may become resistant and very upset. If this is observed, then you may need to end the study early (Benson and Lefton-Grief, 1994).

Analysis of the Study

It is beyond the scope of this book to address how to analyze the study. An SLP who performs MBS studies must be sure she demonstrates competency. Two

Chapter 4: Instrumentation, Devices, and Diagnostic Procedures, continued

helpful documents entitled "Skills Needed by SLPs Providing Services to Dysphagic Patients/Clients" and "Instrumental Diagnostic Procedures for Swallowing" can be obtained from the American Speech-Language-Hearing Association. There are enough differences in children and adults that SLPs who perform studies on children and adults must make sure they are competent with both.

Other Procedures

Manometry

This technique quantifies the strength of contractions of the muscular walls of the gut. It measures the motor activity by measuring strength, speed, and duration of muscle contractions. This is done using intra-luminal pressure transducers. It is not an imaging study. Manometry might be used to measure the pressure in the lower esophageal sphincter to see if it fails to relax, or to see if it has too low a pressure (e.g., allows reflux more easily). Manometry is also used to assess the opening of the upper esophageal sphincter.

Nuclear Scintigraphy

This diagnostic procedure involves swallowing a small amount of radionuclide isotope during the feeding. By obtaining images over a period of time after the material is swallowed, the scan provides information about the kind of reflux occurring, how high the reflux goes in the esophagus, and whether or not it enters the airway. It appears to have a high false positive rate.

pH Probe Monitoring

This procedure is used to assess gastroesophageal reflux. A small sensor similar to an NG tube is placed just above the lower esophageal sphincter to measure the acidity in the esophagus. This probe typically is in place for at least 24 hours. It allows the examiner to know when the episodes of reflux occur so that it can be determined if there is a relationship between the reflux and such things as the child's position, level of activity, when the last meal was eaten, etc.

Bronchoscopy

Bronchoscopy is an endoscopic evaluation of the lower airway and is used to identify abnormalities of the airway. Physicians typically perform bronchoscopy if there is persistent stridor, recurrent pneumonia, wheezing, etc.

Extracorporeal Membrane Oxygenation (ECMO)

ECMO is a process to oxygenate the blood of a patient outside the body. A carotid artery and one of the jugular veins are tied off and the blood is shunted to a lung machine to be oxygenated. The blood is then returned to the circulatory system. The technique is used to support an impaired respiratory system (Mosby, 1994).

ECMO is a complex and costly technique, and is not available at all hospitals, even those with neonatal intensive care units. It is commonly used with near-term infants with persistent pulmonary hypertension due to meconium aspiration, congenital diaphragmatic hernia, sepsis, and respiratory distress.

There are risks associated with this procedure. They include neurological deficits (e.g., neuromotor impairment), sensory impairment (e.g., blindness), developmental impairment, and seizure disorder. The most severe possible risk is death. However, a randomized trial completed in the United Kingdom in 1996 revealed that ECMO appeared to reduce mortality in mature newborns with respiratory failure.

ECMO is not performed on premature infants weighing less than 2000 grams, as they have an increased risk of intracranial hemorrhage (Makhoul et al., 1994). There also appears to be an increase in intracranial hemorrhage when the infant is on ECMO for a longer period of time (Bulas et al., 1996). Agnos (1998) has observed that infants who were placed on ECMO had a weak suck and were disorganized, but responded well to therapeutic techniques.

Monitors

Cardiorespiratory Monitor

This monitor gives a visual display in the form of a graph of the child's respirations and heartbeat. It also provides a numeric value (e.g., 155 beats per minute). The numeric values do not reflect brief changes because they are obtained by averaging activity over a short period of time. That is, the numeric value displayed at any one time reflects an average of what has occurred during the last 10 seconds. The graph reflects temporary changes. This monitor is also very sensitive to movement, and therefore, the values may not be accurate.

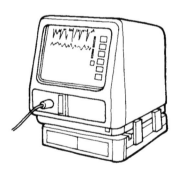

Watching the graph during treatment can help you determine if the child's physiologic state is changing (i.e., reflecting stress). For example, if the infant's respiratory rate increases during feeding, check with the nurse.

Chapter 4: Instrumentation, Devices, and Diagnostic Procedures, continued

Pulse Oximeter

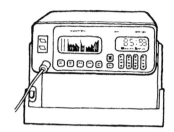

Oximeters monitor the amount of oxygen saturating the capillary blood flow. A sensor is placed on a finger, toe, hand, or foot to measure the percent of oxygen saturation. Wolf (1992) reports that most normal infants maintain a saturation level above 95%. With premature infants, an acceptable rate is usually 90%, but check with the nursing staff to see what the baseline level is. The alarm on the monitor can be set at different levels depending on the desired baseline. Movement, pigmentation of the skin, external light sources, and infrared heating sources can effect oximetry readings.

Watch the monitor for any drop in oxygen saturation below baseline. If oxygen saturation drops during feeding, remove the nipple so the child can breathe. Then consult with the nurse.

Suctioning

Many children with developmental disabilities require suctioning of excess secretions in the oropharynx. Portable suction machines may be used in the home or at school. A tonsil tip or Yankauer suction may be used in the oral cavity. For deep suctioning, sterile techniques are used. A catheter is inserted through the nose into the hypopharynx and trachea. If the child has a tracheostomy, suctioning will be performed through the tracheostomy tube.

Tube Feeding

There are basically five types of tubes that are used to feed infants and children with feeding disorders. Naso-gastric, naso-duodenal, and oro-gastric tubes are used more on a short-term basis. Whereas naso-gastric tubes are often left in place with adults, they are sometimes placed for each feeding with the pediatric population. Percutaneous endoscopic gastrostomy tubes and percutaneous endoscopic jejunostomy tubes are used on a more long-term basis.

Naso-gastric tube (NG tube)

The NG tube is placed through the child's nose into the esophagus with the tip resting in the stomach. Physician practices may vary, with some physicians preferring to leave the NG tube in for several days. Other physicians prefer the tube be changed daily from one nostril to the other or reinserted for each feeding. The tube often has to be taped to the face. This, and the frequent insertion and removal of the tube, can cause the child to develop an aversion to being touched about the face. An infant or child can eat by mouth while an NG tube is in place.

Naso-duodenal tube

This tube is inserted through the nose, but goes past the stomach to the beginning of the small intestine that is called the duodenum. If a child has problems with reflux, this may be the tube chosen by the physician. This allows the formula to be placed in the intestines rather than in the stomach, somewhat reducing the risk of reflux.

Oro-gastric tube

An oro-gastric tube runs from the mouth to the stomach. It is very difficult for the child to eat by mouth with an oro-gastric tube in place. These are almost always removed after each feeding and replaced for the next feeding.

Percutaneous endoscopic gastrostomy tube (PEG tube)

The PEG tube is placed via a surgical procedure through the abdominal wall directly into the stomach. The advantage with the PEG tube is that it can be kept under clothing and the child is less likely to pull at it. There is no tape or aversive stimuli around the face and it can be used on a much longer-term basis.

Percutaneous endoscopic jejunoscopy (PEJ tube)

The PEJ tube is placed similarly to the gastrostomy tube, but the surgery passes through the abdominal wall into the jejunum, which is the beginning of the small intestine past the duodenum. There is a reduced risk of reflux with a PEJ compared to a PEG.

Positioning during tube feeding

Children should not lie flat when receiving tube feedings. Tube feedings should be given at slow enough rates to allow the stomach to empty during the feeding to reduce the risk of vomiting. The child may be positioned prone on a wedge if at high-risk for reflux (See information on GERD in Chapter 2, pages 32-35).

Bolus vs. Continuous

Bolus feedings mean that the formula is given all at once, usually over a period of 15 to 20 minutes. Continuous feedings require the use of a feeding pump and typically are given during the night. The physician decides which is the most appropriate for the child.

Chapter 4: Instrumentation, Devices, and Diagnostic Procedures, continued

Appendix 4-A

Barium Cookie Recipe

Ingredients

1 c. granulated sugar
4 T. butter
1 egg
¼ c. milk
10 T. barium powder (about ¾ c.) (You can get this from the Radiology Dept.)

1 t. vanilla
2 c. flour (all-purpose or whole wheat, sifted)
1 t. baking soda
¼ t. salt

Procedure
Sift the sugar into a large bowl. Beat the butter until soft, gradually adding the sugar. Blend until creamy. In another bowl, combine the egg, milk, and vanilla and beat. Set aside.

In a third bowl, combine the flour, baking soda, barium powder, and salt. Sift the mixture. Add the flour mixture and milk mixture to the butter and sugar, alternating small amounts of each. Beat the batter after each addition. You may need to add extra milk if the batter is too sticky.

Using a teaspoon, place ½-inch portions of dough onto a greased baking sheet. Bake in a preheated oven (375° F) for about nine minutes. Cool before eating. These cookies freeze well.

Optional: Sprinkle each cookie with sugar before baking.

Yield: Approximately 75 cookies

Chapter 4: Instrumentation, Devices, and Diagnostic Procedures, *continued*

References

ASHA. *Skills Needed by SLPs Providing Services to Dysphagic Patients/Clients*, Vol. 32, Supplement 2, 1990, pp. 7-12.

ASHA. *Instrumental Diagnostic Procedures for Swallowing*, Vol. 34, Supplement 7, 1992, pp. 25-33.

Beck, T.J. and Gayler, B.W. "Radiation in Video-Recorded Fluoroscopy." In Jones, B. et al. (eds.) *Normal and Abnormal Swallowing - Imaging and Diagnosis in Therapy*, New York: Springer-Verlag, 1991, pp. 1-6.

Benson, J.E. and Lefton-Greif, M.A. "Videofluoroscopy of Swallowing in Pediatric Patients: A Component of the Total Feeding Evaluation." In Tuchman, D. and Walter, R. (eds.) *Disorders of Feeding and Swallowing in Infants and Children: Pathophysiology, Diagnosis, and Treatment*, San Diego: Singular Publishing Group, Inc., 1994.

Bulas, D.I. et al. "Intercranial Abnormalities in Infants Treated with Extracorporeal Membrane Oxygenation: Update on Sonographic and CT Findings." *American Journal of Neuroradiology*, Vol. 17, No. 2, 1996, pp. 287-294.

Jolley, S.G. et al. "Pharyngeal and Swallowing Disorders in Infants." *Seminars in Pediatric Surgery*, Vol. 4, No. 3, 1997, pp. 157-165.

Linden, P. "Videofluoroscopy in Rehabilitation for Swallowing Dysfunction." *Dysphagia*, Vol. 3, 1989, pp. 189-191.

Logemann, J.A. *Manual for the Videofluorographic Study of Swallowing*, San Diego: College Hill Press, 1986.

Makhoul, I.R. et al. "Predicators of Neonatal Mortality in 1,500-1,999g Premature Infants with Respiratory Failure. Basis for ECMO Therapeutic Trial." *Journal of the American Society for Artificial Organs*, Vol. 40, No. 1, 1994, pp. 27-32.

Marquis, J. and Pressman, H. "Radiologic Assessment of Pediatric Swallowing." In Rosenthal, S. et al. (eds.) *Dysphagia and the Child with Developmental Disabilities: Medical, Clinical and Family Interventions*, San Diego: Singular Publishing Group, Inc., 1995, p. 135.

Mosby's *Medical, Nursing, and Allied Health Dictionary*, 5th ed, St. Louis: Mosby Year Book, Inc., 1998, p. 605.

UK Collaborative ECMO Trial Group. "UK Collaborative Randomized Trial of Neonatal Extracorporeal Membrane Oxygenation." *The Lancet*, Vol. 348, No. 9020, 1996, pp. 75-78.

Wolf, L.F. and Glass, R.P. *Feeding and Swallowing Disorders in Infancy: Assessment and Management*, San Antonio: Therapy Skill Builders, a division of The Psychological Corporation, 1992.

Chapter 5: Treatment of Feeding Disorders

This chapter describes techniques which may be helpful for children of all ages (infant through school age). Some of the information is more applicable to infants than to older children and vice versa. For example, the feeding position of holding a child in front of you works for a six-month-old, but not a five-year-old. Conversely, a technique used to alert a child such as using textured foods would not be appropriate for a four-month-old. Techniques specific to infants are described in more detail in Chapter 6.

Total Oral-Motor Program vs. Isolated Feeding Therapy

Several well-known swallowing specialists (Morris and Klein, 1987; Arvedson and Brodsky, 1997; Alexander, 1987) stress the importance of a total program of oral-motor development over isolated work on feeding. If a total oral-motor approach is used with the child, then oral-motor development becomes the primary goal and feeding becomes the secondary goal. You may not even introduce food and liquid during therapy sessions because there are other ways to address oral-motor goals.

As is the case in many areas of speech and language, there is not a great deal of research to support one particular approach. However, clinical experience supports the fact that the development of positioning, stability, and oral-motor skills does yield better results than directly working on feeding (Morris, 1985). Morris examined the relationship of the development of movements and processes for speech and for feeding. She found three components were essential for developing both speech and feeding skills:

1. An increase in the number and type of oral movements and positions

2. Adding other simple movement patterns and integrating them with previously learned patterns

3. The ability to separate movement of two or more components of the system (e.g., head separate from trunk, mouth separate from head)

Therefore, it appears that the development of movement is essential to the development of early sound production and feeding abilities.

Components of the Total Oral-Motor Approach

Controlling oral-motor skills:	Food presentation changes:
• changing the physical environment and stimuli in the environment • changing the child's position • exercises for the oral mechanism	• texture/temperature • timing • amount/size of bolus

Chapter 5: Treatment of Feeding Disorders, continued

Creating a Conducive Environment in Which the Child is Fed

An environment with too many auditory and visual distractions may make it difficult for the child to respond. It is important to reduce auditory and visual distractions as much as possible. You may want some quiet background music, but you certainly do not want other extraneous noises such as siblings shouting, dogs barking, or sounds of cooking. If the child is overstimulated by these sounds, he will not be able to pay attention to the feeding.

Explore the tastes, textures, and temperatures the child responds to best. There may be some tastes, textures, and temperatures to which the child has an aversive reaction.

Older children who cannot communicate verbally or through augmented means may use nonverbal cues to communicate during mealtime. Pay careful attention to signals provided by the child such as looking away from you as you present the food to him, shaking his head "no," or looking somewhat afraid if you are presenting a drink before he is ready. For children who are using an augmentative or alternative form of communication, be sure to incorporate the use of the system during mealtimes. Include concepts such as *more, stop,* and food choices.

Children need to be in an appropriate state of alertness and attention to experience a successful and pleasant feeding experience. Consider the following tips to help achieve the desired level of alertness and attention with older children for successful feeding:

Mode of Input	Alerting	Calming
Movement/Touch	uneven or rough textures very warm and very cold stimuli light tickles vibration (e.g., electric toothbrush) textured foods cold foods	Be sure child is positioned in a stable way so he is not constantly having to fight to maintain stability during a meal. For hyperactive children, a slow rocking or bouncing movement or even swinging may be helpful. (Try this before the meal.) Use heavier utensils. Use foods and liquids of more thickness and texture. Provide deep pressure to limbs and trunk.

continued

Chapter 5: Treatment of Feeding Disorders, continued

Mode of Input	Alerting	Calming
Taste/Smell	Use foods with very sharp tastes such as sour, bitter, salty, or sweet. (Keep in mind that purchased baby foods have very little salt or sugar added, and therefore, may be too bland to alert older children. You might want to blend the baby food with table food.) herbs and spices any strong and unique smells (e.g., perfume or loose spice tea)	Eliminate foods with sour or bitter tastes.
Visual Input	bright colors shiny objects moving objects movement in the peripheral vision contrast of color and shape	neutral colors dull objects objects that are not moving
Auditory Input	unexpected or loud noises	soft, repetitive sounds music with slow tempo and regular rhythm

Chapter 5: Treatment of Feeding Disorders, continued

Posture and Positioning

Alexander (1998) describes three specific functions related to posture which must be developed for children to be able to eat and drink normally. Alexander indicates that if we simply position a child for postural alignment without helping the child move through postural activity, then we are not helping the child to generalize what we are doing.

Postural activity This is how the body works through the developmental process to get ready to actively control and move against gravity in a coordinated fashion. Postural activity is necessary to establish a postural base.

Postural control This is activation within the system to control posture without the extraneous movement that is seen in younger babies. Older children with developmental disorders may not have achieved postural control and may still need postural activity in order to coordinate respiration and phonation.

Postural alignment This is needed for feeding and swallowing. The components of good postural alignment are:

- neutral head flexion (not chin tuck)

- neck elongation

- stable depressed shoulder girdle

- trunk elongation (proper balance between flexion and extension)

- neutral base at the pelvis (a little anterior tilt at hips)

- 90° hip flexion with feet on a stable surface for weight-bearing

What Alexander describes as postural activity, Rosenthal et al. (1995) describe as preparatory activities. Some preparatory activities may be beneficial before placing the child in the positions described below. Children often benefit from gentle rocking, bouncing, or joint compression activities. If you are working with a physical therapist, ask her to design activities to achieve the following:

- neck elongation and chin tuck (Alexander, 1987)

- balanced muscle tone in trunk and limbs for sitting (Morris, 1987)

- balanced muscle tone and stability in the shoulder girdle (Nelson and DeBeenabib, 1991)

Chapter 5: Treatment of Feeding Disorders, *continued*

It is beyond the scope of this book to fully describe activities designed to improve postural and preparatory activity. There are intensive and in-depth training courses (e.g., Neurodevelopmental Treatment) that provide the needed information and practice to become adept at this. In addition, working closely with a pediatric physical therapist can provide you with information about postural activity and postural control. We will focus our discussion on postural alignment.

Postural Alignment

Appropriate postural alignment for infants may be achieved in one of the following ways:

Hold the infant cradled in one arm.

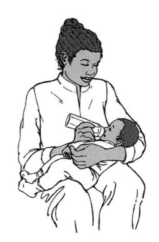

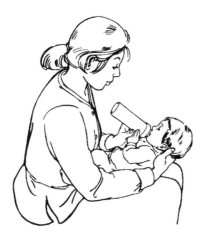

Hold the infant in front of you with your arm and hand supporting the neck and head. This position allows you to have eye contact with the infant.

Sit cross-legged and place the infant on your lap, facing you. Place a pillow under the infant for more support. This position also allows you to have eye contact with the child.

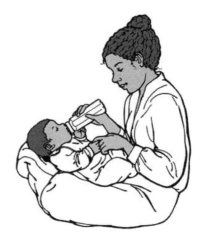

The Source for Pediatric Dysphagia

Chapter 5: Treatment of Feeding Disorders, *continued*

Seat the child beside you. Put your arm around the child so you can use your shoulder and body to help maintain the child's position. Feed the child with your other hand.

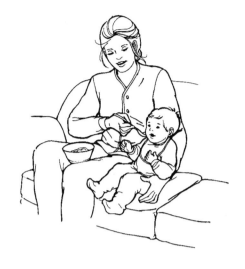

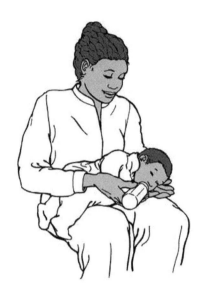

Use a sidelying position to feed the infant. This allows good support for the trunk. If the infant is exhibiting a retracted tongue, this position may help the tongue come forward. You may need to bring the head into slight hyperextension for the child who is having respiratory problems. If the child is having trouble sucking and maintaining a lip seal, you might try greater head flexion.

Use a prone position. This should be done with the shoulders higher than the hips, such as when lying across a wedge. This prone position is helpful because gravity helps the jaw and the tongue fall forward. It may be necessary to place your hand under the child's jaw to provide additional jaw support.

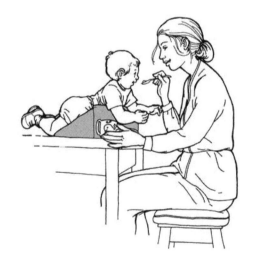

The Source for Pediatric Dysphagia

Chapter 5: Treatment of Feeding Disorders, continued

Relationship of Head and Neck

Pay close attention to the relationship of the head and neck. If the child is in a hyperextended position, it is very difficult to achieve adequate closure of the airway. It also means that the bolus may fall over the back of the tongue before the child is ready to swallow. Neck hyperextension may also lead to tongue protrusion or tongue retraction patterns or excessive jaw movements that can interfere with sucking (Wolf and Glass, 1992). Excessive neck flexion may also impair maintenance of the airway, and therefore, the infant could be vulnerable to airway collapse or apnea (Thatch and Stark, 1979).

Positioning for Hypertonic and Hypotonic Children

With hypertonic children, it is necessary to inhibit increased tone and to facilitate movement of the extremities. The physical therapist can demonstrate ways to do this.

With hypotonic children, you must help the child achieve alignment and stability and maintain upright posture for feeding. This will also help the child gain symmetrical control.

Although an upright position is typically best, there are some children for whom a slightly reclined position may be better for feeding, including some children with the following:

- poor head control

- poor lip closure and tongue thrusting (e.g., lose a lot out the front of the mouth when upright [Tuchman and Walter, 1994])

Keep in mind that placing a child in a reclined position is going to make it more difficult for him to control the bolus in the oral cavity and may put him at risk for aspiration.

Once children are past the bottle feeding stage, you will probably need some kind of seating system to achieve appropriate postural alignment. (For specific examples of equipment, see Chapter 11.)

Oral-Motor Treatment

There are treatment techniques to directly improve oral-motor skills. Some of the techniques address specific problems. The following pages include:

- Descriptions of specific problems that interfere with feeding. These problems are grouped according to association with increased tone, association with decreased tone, or association with either increased or decreased tone.

Chapter 5: Treatment of Feeding Disorders, *continued*

- Charts that identify treatment techniques most helpful for specific problems. The charts are organized by problems associated with increased tone, problems associated with decreased tone, or problems not unique to increased or decreased tone.

- Descriptions of treatment techniques and how to perform them. These techniques may be appropriate for children with increased or decreased tone.

These techniques have been described by Morris and Klein (1987), Arvedson and Brodsky (1993), and Wolf and Glass (1992).

Specific Problems that Interfere with Feeding

Problems Associated with Increased Tone

Jaw Thrust Jaw thrust is the sudden and forceful opening of the jaw. It can be caused or exacerbated by:

- poor sitting position with too much hip extension and posterior pelvic tilt (increases body tension)

- a reaction to an overstimulating environment

- dislocation of the temporomandibular joint which may cause pain if jaw is opened

- hypersensitivity in the mouth (the child thrusts jaw in reaction to stimulation)

Jaw Retraction Jaw retraction is the pulling back of the mandible. It can be caused or exacerbated by:

- poor sitting position with too much hip extension and posterior pelvic tilt (increases body tension)

- a reaction to an overstimulating environment

Note: Jaw retraction occurs with a normal size mandible. Micrognathia, or too small a mandible, may make it look like the jaw is retracted when it is not.

Lip Retraction In lip retraction, the lips pull back in a tight, horizontal line. This interferes with sucking from a bottle, removing food from a spoon or cup, and keeping food in the mouth during chewing. It may be caused or exacerbated by:

Chapter 5: Treatment of Feeding Disorders, continued

- poor sitting position with too much hip extension (increases body tension)
- a reaction to an overstimulating environment

Note: When the child attempts to talk or eat, the lips may appear pursed.

Problems Associated with Decreased Tone

Jaw Clenching Jaw clenching is tight squeezing of the teeth or grinding of the teeth. It can be caused or exacerbated by:

- poor sitting position with too much hip flexion and posterior tilt of the pelvis (increase in body flexion)
- low tone in the trunk and postural instability (causes the child to slump)
- reaction to low tone in the trunk (causes child to clench jaw to keep it from hanging open)
- a reaction to an overstimulating environment
- hypersensitivity in the mouth (causes child to clench teeth in reaction to teeth touching each other)
- child clenching teeth on purpose to keep anything from being stuck into the mouth (or it may be attention seeking)

Jaw Instability Jaw instability results in the jaw shifting from side to side or forward. It may be caused or exacerbated by:

- hypotonic face and trunk

Tongue Thrust Tongue thrust is the forceful protrusion of the tongue out of the mouth. This may be caused or exacerbated by:

- the child's compensation to low tone (pushes tongue forward more forcefully)
- hyperextension of the neck with shoulders retracted (causes an increase in extensor patterns)
- the child's compensation for difficulty breathing (keeping the tongue forward helps the child breathe)

Chapter 5: Treatment of Feeding Disorders, *continued*

- delayed development of tongue lateralization, so the child has to use tongue thrust to move food around in the mouth

Bunchy Tongue A thick, humped tongue can interfere with sucking and forming a bolus. This may be caused or exacerbated by:

- low tone in the mouth

- decreased sensation in the mouth

- damage to cranial nerve XII (can result in decreased movement)

- damage to cranial nerve VII (can result in decreased sensation)

Low Tone in the Cheeks Hypotonia, or low tone in the cheeks, interferes with efficient sucking, bolus formation, and bolus maintenance. It may be caused or exacerbated by:

- low tone in the rest of the body

- decreased sensation in the face and mouth

- damage to cranial nerve VII (can result in facial weakness)

- damage to cranial nerve V (can result in decreased sensation in the face)

Problems Not Unique to Increased or Decreased Tone

Tonic Bite Reflex Tonic bite reflex is when the mandible clenches on an object. It may be caused or exacerbated by:

- poor sitting position with too much hip flexion or extension with posterior pelvic tilt (leads to increased body flexion and tension)

- a reaction to an overstimulating environment

- oral hypersensitivity

- child clenching teeth shut on purpose to keep anything out of his mouth

Chapter 5: Treatment of Feeding Disorders, continued

Oral Hypersensitivity	This is a reaction to stimuli that is much stronger than expected. This can be caused or exacerbated by:

- low threshold to stimulation secondary to neurological damage

- increased postural tone

- overall lack of stimulation that normally occurs when feeding children who are tube fed

- hypersensitive gag

Tongue Retraction   Tongue retraction occurs when the tongue pulls back into the oral cavity. It may be caused or exacerbated by:

- low tone that creates exaggerated extensor movements

- high tone that creates exaggerated extensor movements

- neck hyperextension and shoulder retraction

Note: Children with Pierre Robin and micrognathia have their tongue retracted into the airway. Children with a hard palate cleft may pull tongue back to fill the opening.

Limited Tongue Movement   Limited tongue movement can be seen in eating and when mouthing toys. It may be caused or exacerbated by:

- high tone (causes tongue to be stiff)

- low tone (causes tongue to be floppy)

- flaccid tongue secondary to cranial nerve XII damage

Limited Upper Lip Movement   Limited upper lip movement can be seen in eating, when mouthing toys, or making sounds. It may be caused or exacerbated by:

- high tone (causes lips and cheeks to be stiff)

- low tone (causes lips and cheeks to be floppy)

- facial weakness secondary to cranial nerve VII damage

- decreased facial sensations secondary to cranial nerve V damage

The Source for Pediatric Dysphagia

Chapter 5: Treatment of Feeding Disorders, *continued*

Hyperactive Gag This is an exaggerated response to stimulation in the mouth. It may be caused or exacerbated by:

- lowered threshold to stimuli secondary to neurological damage

- decreased experience with stimuli in the mouth related to tube feeding

The charts on the following pages (pages 140-146) show various techniques and how they may serve more than one purpose. Descriptions of the treatment techniques indicated in the charts are described in greater detail on pages 146-153.

Chapter 5: Treatment of Feeding Disorders, continued

Treatment Techniques for Problems Associated with Increased Tone

Technique	Components *	Jaw Thrust	Jaw Retraction	Lip Retraction
better sitting posture	trunk and pelvis aligned shoulders forward neck elongated chin tuck (capital flexion)	X	X	X
examine sensory input to child	reduce visual input to child provide quiet background soothing music explore tastes, textures, temperatures	X	X	X
position prone	shoulders higher than hips gravity helps jaw and tongue fall forward hand under jaw	X	X	
reduce hypersensitivity to contact with teeth	firm pressure to face, gums, teeth help maintain jaw closure to increase stability	X		
increase sensory input to tongue through toothbrushing	fingers and toys in mouth first rub all surfaces in mouth proceed carefully beginning toothbrush sets brush all surfaces introduce tastes on brushes	X		
playful activities to maintain jaw closure	clench cloth between teeth hold straw between teeth	X		
vibrations on face and cheeks	vibrate/shake cheeks with index and middle finger vibrate from nose down through upper lip			X

* For more detailed information, see descriptions beginning on page 146.

continued

Chapter 5: Treatment of Feeding Disorders, *continued*

Technique	Components	Jaw Thrust	Jaw Retraction	Lip Retraction
facial molding	wipe with cloth toward mouth			X
help achieve jaw closure	hand on jaw from front or back	X		

Chapter 5: Treatment of Feeding Disorders, continued

Treatment Techniques for Problems Associated with Decreased Tone

Technique	Components *	Jaw Clench	Jaw Instability	Tongue Thrust	Bunchy Tongue	Low Tone Cheek
better sitting posture	trunk and pelvis aligned shoulders forward neck elongated chin tuck (capital flexion)	X		X		
position prone	shoulders higher than hips gravity helps jaw and tongue fall forward hand under jaw	X				
reduce hypersensitivity to contact with teeth	firm pressure to face, gums, and teeth help maintain jaw closure to increase stability	X				
increase sensory input to tongue through toothbrushing	fingers and toys in mouth first rub all surfaces in mouth proceed carefully small, soft-bristled toothbrushes brush all surfaces introduce tastes on brushes	X			X	
playful activities to maintain jaw closure	clench cloth between teeth hold straw between teeth		X			
increase postural tone in trunk	consult with PT	X	X	X	X	X

* For more detailed information, see descriptions beginning on page 146.

continued

Chapter 5: Treatment of Feeding Disorders, continued

Technique	Components	Jaw Clench	Jaw Instability	Tongue Thrust	Bunchy Tongue	Low Tone Cheek
help achieve jaw closure	hand on jaw from front or back		X	X		
tactile and proprioceptive stimulation of jaw muscles	tap cheeks and TMJ in rhythmic fashion		X			X
move child to textured foods	develop tongue and cheek movements develop munching move from suckle to suck				X	
create tongue bowl	even pressure with bowl of spoon on tongue can use some vibration			X		
vibrations to tongue and oral cavity	electric toothbrush other vibratory source				X	
increase tongue stability for more forward movement	chin tuck position tap under chin on base of tongue				X	
straw drinking	use squeeze bottle reduce assistance to lips only small portions of straw in mouth					X
quick stretch	over area of masseter and buccinator		X			X

Chapter 5: Treatment of Feeding Disorders, *continued*

Treatment Techniques for Problems Not Unique to Increased or Decreased Tone

Technique	Components *	Tonic Bite Reflex	Oral Hypersensitivity	Tongue Retraction	Limited Tongue Movement	Limited Upper Lip Movement	Hyperactive Gag
better sitting posture	trunk and pelvis aligned shoulders forward neck elongated chin tuck (capital flexion)	X					
position prone	shoulders higher than hips gravity helps jaw and tongue fall forward hand under jaw			X			
reduce hyper-sensitivity to contact with teeth	firm pressure to face, gums, teeth help maintain jaw closure to increase stability	X	X				X
increase sensory input to tongue through toothbrushing	fingers and toys in mouth first rub all surfaces in mouth proceed carefully beginning toothbrush sets brush all surfaces introduce tastes on brushes	X	X		X		X
vibrations on face and cheeks	vibrate/shake cheeks with index and middle finger vibrate from nose down through upper lip					X	

* For more detailed information, see descriptions beginning on page 146.

continued

The Source for Pediatric Dysphagia

Chapter 5: Treatment of Feeding Disorders, continued

Technique	Components	Tonic Bite Reflex	Oral Hypersensitivity	Tongue Retraction	Limited Tongue Movement	Limited Upper Lip Movement	Hyperactive Gag
increase postural tone in the trunk	consult with PT			X	X	X	
tactile and proprioceptive stimulation of jaw muscles	tap cheeks and TMJ in rhythmic fashion					X	
vibrations to tongue and oral cavity	electric toothbrush other vibratory source		X		X		X
increase tongue stability for more forward movement	chin tuck position tap under chin on base of tongue			X	X		
vibration of center of tongue to flatten it	enter mouth from the side downward vibration on center of tongue lateral vibrations			X	X		
vibrations to upper lip	vibratory source					X	
quick stretch	forefinger and middle finger on upper lip provide quick stretch out					X	
increase sensory input to upper lip	explore toys and/or variety of tastes on lips					X	

continued

The Source for Pediatric Dysphagia

Chapter 5: Treatment of Feeding Disorders, continued

Technique	Components	Tonic Bite Reflex	Oral Hypersensitivity	Tongue Retraction	Limited Tongue Movement	Limited Upper Lip Movement	Hyperactive Gag
increase control of upper lip through straw drinking	squeeze bottles thicker liquids longer straws					X	
desensitize tongue	firm downward pressure gradually move back head flexion		X				X
grading stimuli	carefully monitor child's response grade: area of body, type of texture		X				

Description of Treatment Techniques

The following text and illustrations provide more information about how to perform the techniques listed on the previous charts.

Reducing Hypersensitivity to Contact with Teeth

Provide firm pressure to the face first. As the child begins to tolerate your touch, work your way into the child's mouth to provide firm pressure to the gums or to the teeth. Enter the child's mouth from the side rather than directly from the front. Start by providing firm pressure on the outer gum ridge at the midline and moving toward the back of the mouth. Repeat this several times on the upper and lower gums. Be sure to pause in between to allow the child to swallow. Try this first on the lateral surfaces and then on the superior surfaces. Provide jaw support to give the child increased jaw stability during these activities. (See the illustrations on page 147.)

Chapter 5: Treatment of Feeding Disorders, continued

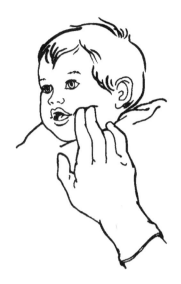 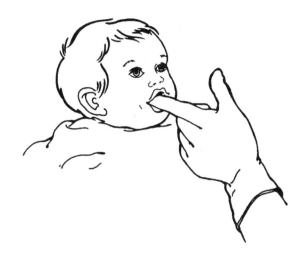

Note: When you are working with activities designed to reduce tonic bite reflex, there is the possibility you will be bitten. Do not try to pull your finger out, as this will only increase the tonic bite. Try to maintain a calm demeanor. If you panic, you will increase the child's overall body tension and tone and will again strengthen the tonic bite. Try to rock and calm the child to eliminate the tonic bite. Most children will open their mouths if their heads are hyperextended, so you might try changing the child to that position.

If these techniques don't work, and there is another person around, have her place her thumbs on both sides of the child's jaw on the TMJ joint and apply inward pressure on the joint to release the bite. In a severe case, you can usually get a child to release the bite by blowing a puff of air in the child's face, sprinkling water in the child's face, or even holding the child's nose. Do not use these latter techniques unless it is absolutely necessary.

Increase Sensory Input to Tongue Through Toothbrushing

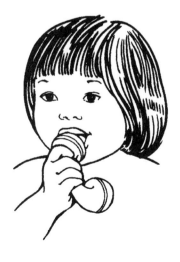

Encourage the child to place his fingers and toys in his mouth first before attempting any toothbrushing. Have the child get used to rubbing all surfaces in his mouth, including the chewing surfaces, inside the cheeks, lateral borders of the tongue, and the top of the tongue.

Carefully introduce toothbrushing. Start along the sides of the child's tongue on the lateral borders, and gradually work toward the midline of the tongue. This may take several sessions. Begin the toothbrushing with a piece of terry cloth wrapped around your finger and then move through a series of other brushes. NUK® provides a gradual increase in textures.

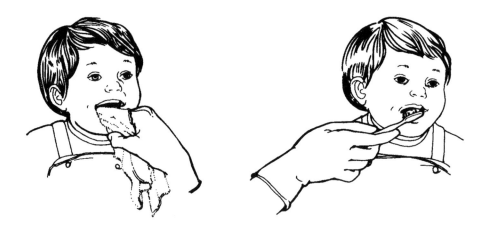

Help Maintain Jaw Closure

Have the child hold a piece of terry cloth or a small toy in his mouth as you shake it back and forth. Time how long the child can maintain jaw closure with the object in his mouth.

Vibrations on Face and Cheeks

Vibrations on the face and cheeks can occur in two ways. Put your index finger inside the child's mouth in the buccal cavity and your middle finger on the exterior surface of the cheek. This way, you have the child's cheek lightly pinched between your forefinger and your middle finger. Use a very quick shaking or vibration of the fingers as you pull the cheek forward and pull your finger out of the child's mouth.

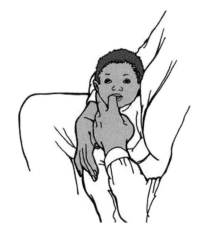

Chapter 5: Treatment of Feeding Disorders, continued

You can also place your index finger and middle finger on either side of the bridge of the child's nose. Use a very quick vibrating motion to pull and work down all the way through the upper lip. Do not stop until you've come to the corner of the upper lip to help the child move the lip down.

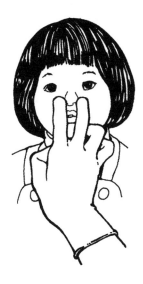 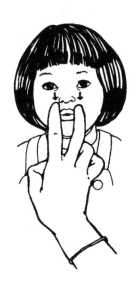

Facial Molding

Wipe the child's face with a cloth. Wipe from the outer cheek (in front of the ear) forward toward the lips. Wipe from the bottom of the chin up towards the lips. Use a firm, gentle pressure. If you don't have a warm cloth or terry cloth, you can use your hands. After the molding takes place, follow with a functional activity such as non-nutritive sucking on a pacifier, nipple, or with some cup or spoon-feeding. Provide facial molding on both sides of the child's face, either alternating sides or to both sides at the same time.

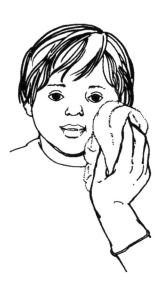

Chapter 5: Treatment of Feeding Disorders, continued

Help Achieve Jaw Closure

Children with jaw thrust or jaw instability have difficulty maintaining jaw closure. Provide support to the child, either from the side or from the front.

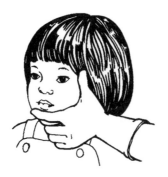
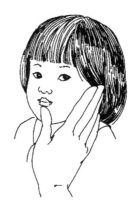

Tactile and Proprioceptive Stimulation of the Jaw Muscles

Tap in a rhythmic fashion on the temporo-mandibular joint to increase tone in the cheeks which may also help with better lip movement. You can also tap on the child's cheeks and move toward the lips. Patting and stroking can also be used.

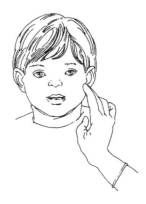

Move to More Textured Foods

When more textured foods are added, the child may not have to use as much tongue protrusion to move the bolus backward. This helps the child develop some up-and-down tongue movements and early munching patterns as food changes are introduced.

Create a Tongue Bowl

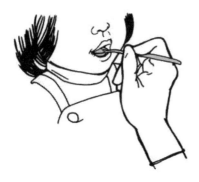

Use a spoon with a fairly flat, small bowl so it's not too large for the child's tongue. Put the spoon in the middle of the child's tongue and press down evenly. Vibrate the spoon. As you remove the spoon, encourage the child to close her lips to help take the food off the spoon. Remind the child to keep the food in the middle of her tongue.

Vibrations to Tongue and Oral Cavity

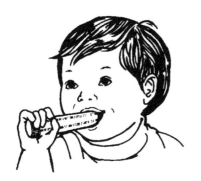

Use a small battery-operated, hand-held vibrator or a vibrating toothbrush. Encourage the child to hold the vibrator and to begin to stimulate the lateral chewing surfaces and gums inside of the cheek first. Gradually work toward the midline of the tongue.

Increase Tongue Stability for More Forward Movement of the Tongue

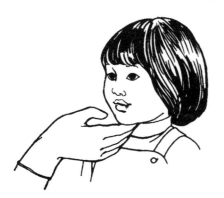

Help the child sit with her neck elongated and in the chin-tucked position. Tap upward on the base of the child's tongue muscle under the chin.

Vibrations of Center of Tongue

First reduce hypertonicity in the neck and shoulder girdle. Consult with the physical therapist for specific techniques. Then enter the child's mouth from the side with your finger. Move toward the center of the child's tongue. Shake your finger with a fine vibration.

Vibrations to Upper Lip

After reducing hypertonicity in the neck and shoulder girdle, put your index finger and middle finger on either side of the base of the child's nose and vibrate downward toward the bottom of the upper lip. Make sure you move your fingers down through the lip.

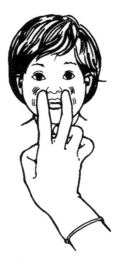

Chapter 5: Treatment of Feeding Disorders, *continued*

Increased Sensory Input to Upper Lip

Encourage the child to provide vibration to his upper lip. Provide other stimulation such as ice, spicy or sour foods, and/or different textures on the upper lip to increase sensation.

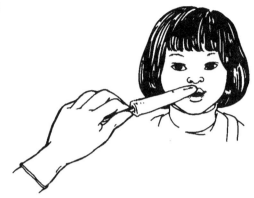

Increased Control of Upper Lips Through Straw Drinking

Begin with a squeeze bottle with a straw so you can squeeze some of the material into the straw to help the child. Gradually squeeze less and make the child suck more. You may have to provide some lip support during this activity. Move toward thicker liquids and longer straws which both require that the child use increased lip activity for better sucking.

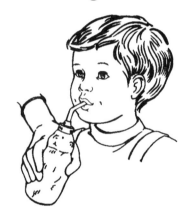

Quick Stretch

Place your index finger and middle finger on the upper lip immediately below the nose. Give several quick stretches out toward the corner of the lips. This stretch can also be done over the masseter for improved jaw stability and to increase tone in the cheeks. The stretch should follow the direction of the muscle.

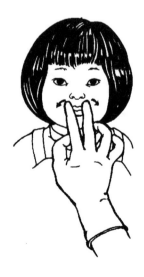
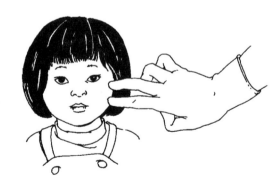

Chapter 5: Treatment of Feeding Disorders, continued

Desensitizing the Tongue

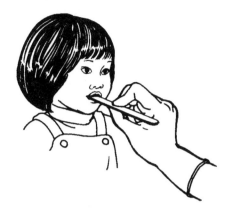

To reduce oral hypersensitivity and hyperactive gag, place your finger, toy, spoon, tongue blade, etc. on the very front of the child's tongue and provide firm pressure. Gradually move it slowly back in the child's mouth with firm pressure each step along the way. If the child starts to gag, help him close his mouth to stop the gag reflex.

Grading Stimuli

For children with oral hypersensitivity, you may need to grade the stimuli you present to the child. This means gradually working up to more aversive stimuli. Carefully monitor the child's response and back off when you can tell the child is becoming stressed.

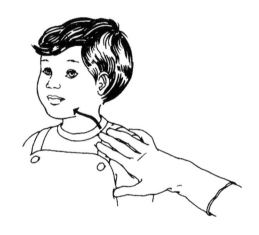

Stimuli can be graded according to the area of the body you are working on. Typically children are more comfortable if you start away from the mouth. Some children need you to start on the hands, arms, and trunk of the body before you work your way up to the face.

The kind of tactile stimulation can also be graded. You can start with very smooth textures and move to rougher and even prickly textures.

You can also grade the amount of pressure provided, starting with a very firm touch and moving to a light touch.

Chapter 5: Treatment of Feeding Disorders, *continued*

Food Presentation

Transitional Feeding

Children typically continue bottle- or breast-feeding until four to six months of age. At that point, the child is usually ready to begin what is termed *transitional feeding*. This means that foods on a spoon will be introduced as well as drinking from a cup.

As noted in Chapter 1 on normal development, these changes in feeding behaviors coincide with the development of specific motor skills such as improved sitting posture and better hand coordination. Children experiencing developmental delays or with developmental disorders may not be ready for transitional feeding at the chronological age of four to six months. Transitional feeding may not occur until the child is at the four- to six-month level developmentally, even though he may be chronologically older.

Spoon Feeding

Children are typically ready to begin spoon feeding at about four to six months of age. Initial trials with a spoon actually resemble sucking food from the spoon (Arvedson and Brodsky, 1993). This sucking motion is different from the sucking motion a child uses on a nipple. To achieve effective spoon feeding for children with dysphagia, it is important NOT to fall into a pattern that is used by caregivers of normal young infants when they begin spoon feeding. That typical pattern is for the pureed food to be scraped off onto the child's upper gum. The child then uses a suckling (enhanced tongue thrusting) pattern which pushes most of the food out of the mouth. The caregiver then scrapes the food off the child's chin and puts it back in the child's mouth. This pattern will not help children with feeding disorders develop a more mature pattern of spoon feeding.

Place the spoon midline on the child's tongue and apply downward pressure. This should encourage lip closure. It also deposits the food at midline where the child will have a better chance of forming a bolus. The child may then use some up-and-down sucking movements instead of a suckling pattern. You may also need to provide external jaw and/or lip support and may also need to provide stimulation to the upper lip to help achieve movement of the upper lip for closure. Begin spoon feeding with smooth, runny, pureed textures. Then introduce foods with other textures and tastes. It is best to introduce only one change at a time (i.e., If you are introducing a new texture, do not introduce a new taste at the same time). A sample recommended sequence of introducing changes is as follows:

1. Introduce runny, pureed peaches.

2. Introduce runny, pureed pears thinned with fruit juice (taste change only).

The Source for Pediatric Dysphagia

Chapter 5: Treatment of Feeding Disorders, *continued*

3. After several days of acceptance of runny pears, introduce pears with some texture (i.e., thicker pureed which hasn't been thinned) (texture change only).

4. Present pears which have been mashed with a fork (texture change only).

5. Give actual small bites of pear (texture change only).

Be sure to allow the child plenty of time (several days) to get used to the change you've introduced before moving to the next step. The most difficult foods for the child to handle will be those with mixed consistencies, such as:

- cereal with milk
- congealed salads (e.g., Jell-O®)
- fruit cocktail
- fruits in juice or syrup
- green beans
- lettuce (salads)
- peas
- stewed tomatoes
- vegetables not drained

If a child has demonstrated oral hypersensitivity, she usually prefers that you present a larger piece of food of the same consistency (e.g., graham crackers or vanilla wafers) rather than foods of two consistencies (e.g., cookie with chocolate chips or cereal in milk).

Give careful consideration to the bite size that is appropriate for the child. You may want to put only a small amount of food on the front of the spoon so that you can control where you deposit the food on the child's tongue.

Be sure to provide jaw support and lower lip support as you withdraw the spoon, especially if the child doesn't use active lip movement to close his mouth. This way, the child will be less likely to push the food out of his mouth.

Cup Drinking

When introducing cup drinking, it is important to choose the right cup. (See Chapter 11.) An appropriate cup typically has a very wide mouth and narrow base or is a cut-out cup which allows the cup to be tipped up without the child's neck going into hyperextension.

Make sure the child's head is appropriately positioned. Place the cup on the child's lower lip, not on his teeth or gums. Provide jaw support. As you tilt the cup, make sure you tilt the cup so the liquid just touches the child's upper lip. This way the child is encouraged to use his lips to draw the liquid into his mouth (Mueller, 1987).

Chapter 5: Treatment of Feeding Disorders, continued

Many feeding specialists advise against using a cup with a spout because they feel it tends to promote a suckling motion rather than mature patterns of cup drinking (Mueller, 1987; Arvedson and Brodsky, 1993). The chart below summarizes Alexander's (1987) description of skills typically developed by children to provide stability needed for cup drinking.

Age	How Child Stabilizes for Cup Drinking
6 months	Lower lip moves up and out to stabilize the cup. It also provides a base for downward movement of the upper lip to help draw liquid in from the cup.
10 months	Tongue protrusion. Also demonstrates an upward and forward motion of the lower lip under the rim of the cup to stabilize the cup.
12-15 months	Biting the cup with active lip closure.

Alexander indicates that coordinated jaw stabilization may not be seen consistently in children until two years of age. We may expect children with developmental disorders to follow this same pattern of development for jaw stabilization using cup drinking.

When children are introduced to cup drinking, they may be startled by the quick flow of a large amount of liquid from a cup as opposed to the very controlled and small amounts they are used to getting from the nipple. Therefore, many children with feeding disorders will do better if you introduce thickened liquids first. These will flow more slowly into the mouth and allow the child to get better control. The thickened liquids may be those which are naturally thick (e.g., nectars), thickened with a commercial thickener (e.g., Thick-It®), or by mixing juice with pureed fruit of the same flavor.

Morris and Klein (1987) suggest that for older children with physical disabilities, more appropriate thickened drinks may include milkshakes, fruit smoothees, or other fruits and vegetables that have been liquified in a blender.

Straw Drinking

Normal children show great variability in when they develop the ability to suck through a straw. This may occur anywhere from one to three years of age (Arvedson and Brodsky, 1993). Straw drinking should not be introduced until the child has demonstrated coordinated ability to drink from a cup.

As noted earlier in this chapter, straw drinking is a technique that can be used to increase lip movement. Mueller (1987) and others suggest that you begin straw drinking by using a polyester tube that is thick walled and has a very small opening such as aquarium tubing. This will allow the child to get some liquid without a very forceful suck. Morris and Klein (1987) describe putting the straw inside a squeeze condiment bottle so a squeezing motion can be used to help the child draw liquid up through the straw. The tubing has to fit tightly in the spout or no suction will be created to allow liquid to be squeezed up into the straw.

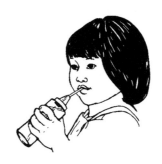

Another way to teach children to drink from a straw is to put a straw into some liquid. Put your finger on the top of the straw to hold some liquid in the straw. Place the other end of the straw in the child's mouth and let him suck as you take your finger off the top of the straw.

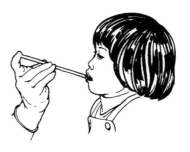

Chewing

To encourage chewing, place the food on the lateral chewing surfaces (i.e., the side teeth, not the back molars). Try foods that are easily chewed and softened with saliva (e.g., graham crackers, vanilla wafers). Avoid foods that fall apart into pieces (e.g., pretzels) or food which doesn't dissolve well (e.g., bread). A gradual transition of food types should be made to develop chewing similar to that described for advancing spoon feeding (pages 154-155).

Do not introduce foods with mixed consistencies until the child shows coordinated use of chewing. This is usually the last kind of texture to introduce. Be sure you do not always place the food on the same side in the child's mouth, but alternate the bites on either of the lateral surfaces. Children following normal development probably develop a mature rotary chew between 24 months of age (Morris and Klein, 1987) and 36 months of age (Alexander, 1987).

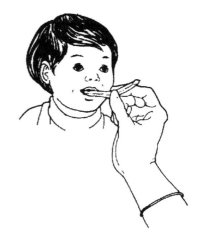

Arvedson and Brodsky (1993) advise using foods that have a long, thin shape (e.g., French fries, pieces of cheese, freshly cooked potato). These allow the feeder to hold on to the food and move the food between the chewing surfaces as needed. The child must learn how to move food from the middle of the tongue to the lateral chewing surfaces.

Chapter 5: Treatment of Feeding Disorders, continued

After the child shows an ability to munch and chew food that is placed directly on the chewing surfaces, put the piece of food on the midline of the tongue to see if the child can independently lateralize it to the chewing surfaces.

The child also needs to be able to move food from one lateral chewing surface, through midline, to the other lateral chewing surface. You may have to help the child understand what you mean by literally moving the food from one side of the child's mouth to the other (i.e., hold a long piece of food and move it for the child).

Biting

A more advanced skill related to chewing is to be able to bite through food presented at the front of the mouth. Do not introduce this until the child is able to move a piece of food from midline to a lateral chewing surface. If introduced before then, the child will simply bite the food and leave it on his tongue. He will be unable to move it to the lateral chewing surfaces. You can, however, allow the child to bite the food and then help move it to the lateral chewing surface.

Mueller (1987) states that you can help a child get the idea of biting by pulling slightly on the food you are placing between the lateral chewing surfaces or by scraping a crusty food on the side of the child's teeth before putting it between his teeth.

Foods with More Texture

Alexander (1987) indicates that there are advantages to introducing foods with more texture for children with cerebral palsy. She states that children with incoordination and delay in the oral stage have a higher potential to aspirate and choke with thin liquids or runny foods than they do with semi-solids or thickened liquids. She also reports that introducing solid foods may improve tongue lateralization and up-and-down jaw movement and may decrease the strength of the gag response. It may also help to develop more active tongue-jaw and cheek-lip movements during chewing and biting. However, if the child has pharyngeal dysphagia, he may have increased residue with thick or sticky foods and therefore may not do as well.

Chapter 5: Treatment of Feeding Disorders, continued

References

Alexander, R. "Oral-Motor and Feeding/Swallowing Function in the Young Child: Assessment and Intervention Strategies." Presentation at Illinois Speech-Language-Hearing Association, Chicago, 1998.

Alexander, R. "Oral-Motor Treatments for Infants and Young Children with Cerebral Palsy." *Seminars in Speech and Language*, Vol. 8, 1987, pp. 87-100.

Alexander, R. "Pre-speech and Feeding Development." In McDonald, E. (ed.) *Treating Cerebral Palsy: For Clinicians By Clinicians*, Austin, TX: Pro-Ed, 1987, pp. 133-152.

Arvedson, J. and Brodsky, L. *Pediatric Swallowing and Feeding: Assessment and Management*, San Diego: Singular Publishing Group, Inc., 1993.

Arvedson, J. et al. "Anatomy, Embryology, and Physiology." In Arvedson, J. and Brodsky, L. (eds.) *Pediatric Swallowing and Feeding: Assessment and Management*, San Diego: Singular Publishing Group, Inc., 1993, pp. 5-12.

Brazelton, T.B. *Neonatal Behavioral Assessment Scale*, Philadelphia: J.D. Lippincott Company, 1984.

Finnie, N. *Handling the Young Cerebral Palsy Child at Home*, 7th ed., New York: E.P. Dutton, 1987.

Griggs, C.A. et al. "Videofluoroscopic Investigation of Feeding Disorders in Children with Multiple Handicaps." *Developmental Medicine and Child Neurology*, Vol. 31, 1989, pp. 303-308.

Harris, M. "Oral-Motor Management of the High Risk Neonate." *Occupational Therapy in Pediatrics*, Vol. 6, 1986, pp. 231-253.

Helfrich-Miller, K.R. et al. "Dysphagia: Its Treatment in the Profoundly Retarded Patient with Cerebral Palsy." *Archives of Physical Medicine and Rehabilitation*, Vol. 67, 1986, pp. 520-525.

Miller, H.D. and Anderson, G.C. "Non-nutritive Sucking: Effects on Crying and Heart Rate on Intubated Infants Requiring Assisted Mechanical Ventilation." *Nursing Research*, Vol. 42, No. 5, 1993, pp. 305-307.

Morris, S.E. "Developmental Implications for the Management of Feeding Problems in Neurologically-Impaired Infants." *Seminars in Speech and Language*, Vol. 6, 1985, pp. 293-315.

Morris, S.E. "Therapy for the Child with Cerebral Palsy: Interacting Framework." *Seminars in Speech and Language*, Vol. 8, 1987, pp. 71-86.

Morris, S.E. and Klein, M.D. *Pre-Feeding Skills: A Comprehensive Resource for Feeding Development*, San Antonio: Therapy Skill Builders, a division of The Psychological Corporation, 1987.

Mueller, H. "Feeding." In Finnie, N. (ed.) *Handling the Young Cerebral Palsy Child at Home*, 7th ed., New York: E.P. Dutton, 1987.

Chapter 5: Treatment of Feeding Disorders, continued

Nelson, C.A. and DeBeenabib, R.M. "Sensory Preparation of the Oral-motor Area." In Langley, M.B. and Lombardino, L.J. (eds.) *Neurodevelopmental Strategies for Managing Communications Disorders in Children with Severe Motor Dysfunction*, Austin, TX: Pro-Ed, 1991, pp. 131-158.

Rosenthal, S. et al. *Dysphagia and the Child with Developmental Disabilities: Medical, Clinical, and Family Interventions*, San Diego: Singular Publishing Group, Inc., 1995.

Thatch, B.T. and Stark, A.R. "Spontaneous Neck Flexion In and Airway Obstruction During Apneic Spells in Pre-Term Infants." *The Journal of Pediatrics*, Vol. 94, 1979, pp. 275-281.

Tuchman, D. and Walter, R. *Disorders of Feeding and Swallowing in Infants and Children: Pathophysiology, Diagnosis, and Treatment*, San Diego: Singular Publishing Group, Inc., 1994.

Wolf, L.F. and Glass R.P. *Feeding and Swallowing Disorders in Infancy: Assessment and Management*, San Antonio: Therapy Skill Builders, a division of The Psychological Corporation, 1992, p. 30.

Chapter 6: Treatment Techniques for Infants

Working with infants with feeding disorders presents a special set of challenges. SLPs may be called in to the neonatal intensive care unit (NICU) to work with premature infants or infants with multiple medical problems. We may be consulted on full-term infants who are a few days old and exhibiting "failure to thrive" (e.g., the child has not developed a good suck or has not latched on well for breast-feeding and the mother is becoming frustrated at her inability to nourish her child). Older babies (months old) may continue to experience feeding difficulties after being discharged from the hospital.

Many of the techniques described in Chapter 5 are applicable to infants. For example, information provided on posture and positioning is important to consider when treating infants. Techniques such as facial molding, vibrations to cheeks, and increasing sensory input (among others) are useful with infants.

This chapter provides more in-depth information about the following topics:

- Paying attention to infant's signals during feeding and responding to these signals

- Tips to calm or alert a baby

- Specific techniques for increasing suck as children are moved from non-oral to oral feeding

- Techniques to improve coordination of sucking, swallowing, and breathing

- Treatment for specific problems in the pharyngeal phase

Distress Signals During Feeding

Infants will signal distress during feeding in a variety of ways. You need to be vigilant in watching for these signs of distress and respond appropriately. Distress signals may include:

Signs of Moderate Distress

- sighing
- yawning
- sneezing
- sweating
- hiccuping
- trembling (jaw/limb)
- startling
- gasping
- facial grimacing
- falling asleep
- squirming
- averting gaze
- straining
- bowel movement
- multiple swallows
- increasing hypertonicity or hypotonicity

Chapter 6: Treatment Techniques for Infants, *continued*

Signs of Major Distress

- coughing
- choking
- spitting up
- gagging
- color change
- respiratory pauses or breath holding
- irregular respiration
- arching back
- bradycardia

(Arvedson and Brodsky, 1993; Morris and Klein, 1987; Agnos, 1998)

Harris (1986) describes two problems infants may demonstrate when becoming functional nipple feeders.

1. Lackadaisical: These infants suck well on a finger or pacifier, but then demonstrate a weak or very dysrhythmic suck with a nipple. During a real feeding, the infant may appear disinterested, may fall asleep, or may even push the nipple away.

2. Aversive: These infants may not even use coordinated non-nutritive sucking on a finger or pacifier. In real feeds, the infant takes a few sucks and then squirms, hyperextends, and arches the body.

Assessing State of Alertness

States of Alertness
Brazelton (1984)

State 1: Deep Sleep: Infant is asleep with a regular breathing pattern. Eyes are closed. No eye movement.
State 2: Light Sleep: Eyes are closed though eye movements may be seen below the lids. Some low-level motor activity may be present.
State 3: Drowsy or Semi-dozing: Eyes are open, but very heavy lidded, or eyes are closed with eyelids fluttering.
State 4: Quiet Alert: Infant is focused on stimulus with a bright look. Motor activity is minimal.
State 5: Active Alert: There is a lot of motor activity including movement of the extremities. There may be brief fussy periods.
State 6: Crying: Infant is crying intensely.

Wolf and Glass (1992) state that feeding may take place during State 3 (drowsy or semi-dozing), State 4 (quiet alert), or State 5 (active alert). They point out that it is important to determine in which state a particular infant is most successful with feeding. For instance, they indicate that a hypersensitive baby who is very disorganized may do better with feeding when she is in a drowsy state than when

Chapter 6: Treatment Techniques for Infants, *continued*

she is in an active alert state. Conversely, a very sleepy baby may only take an adequate amount when she has been made alert. This optimal level of alertness has to be achieved and then maintained throughout the feeding.

The most important time you spend with the baby is before you begin feeding. This time should be used to help the baby achieve the optimal level of alertness for feeding. It may take careful observation of the baby and information from the nurse or caregiver to determine if you need to arouse/alert or calm/soothe the baby before beginning feeding.

The chart below summarizes techniques described by Wolf and Glass and others for alerting or calming the infant. Alerting or calming may be accomplished through the use of movement, auditory stimuli, or tactile stimuli. These techniques may be used before you begin feeding the infant. It may also be necessary during feeding to use the alerting techniques if the infant becomes sleepy or the calming techniques if the infant begins to signal distress.

Achieving Appropriate State

Type of Stimulation	Alerting	Calming
Movement	• Pick the baby up and rock the baby from side to side. • Do not use a rhythmical motion as it will cause the baby to be less alert. • If you firmly support the baby's head, you can use an up-and-down movement.	• Swaddle the baby and use a rhythmic vertical bouncing movement. • Make sure all movement is in a rhythmic manner. • Try rocking, bouncing, or jiggling the baby while standing.
Auditory	• Talk to the baby with varying pitches, volumes, and rhythms. • Music may improve arousal.	• Reduce auditory input to the baby; sometimes not talking to the baby may provide a calming effect. • You can use white noise to block out other sound. • Morris and Klein (1987) describe *hemi-sync music* (i.e., music with a rhythmic background) to provide a calming effect.

continued

Chapter 6: Treatment Techniques for Infants, *continued*

Type of Stimulation	Alerting	Calming
Tactile	• Tickling or light touching on the palms or soles of feet, massaging palms of hands, soles of feet, or crown of head can maintain an alert state. • Put a cool washcloth on the baby's face. • Change the baby's clothes or diapers or unwrap the baby so the baby is not too warm. With very ill infants or infants in the NICU, it is important not to change the temperature too drastically. • Elicit rooting. • Interact with the baby face-to-face.	• Swaddling babies usually provides a very calming effect as it helps the baby feel secure. In addition, the deep pressure provided by the blankets may help the child integrate sensory input. • Reposition the infant by pulling the infant's arms and shoulders slightly forward to midline and slightly flexing the baby's hips. • Try placing a small rolled-up washcloth beneath the infant's feet for the baby to grab with her toes to provide additional calming. Make sure the baby maintains a flexed position. • Provide firm, gentle pressure to the sides of the infant's rib cage. • Non-nutritive sucking

Developing Oral-Motor and Suck-Swallow Skills

Children who are being tube fed often do not develop sucking and swallowing skills to manage their own secretions.

Infants may experience all of the problems described in Chapter 5 such as jaw thrust, tongue retraction, oral hypersensitivity, etc. What follows is a description of problems that may significantly interfere with an adequate suck. The treatment techniques may be particularly useful with very young infants (Wolf and Glass, 1992; Agnos, 1998).

Note: If the problems described in the chart are due to reduced oral-motor skills, then techniques described in Chapter 5 should be addressed. Only additional techniques are listed in the chart.

Chapter 6: Treatment Techniques for Infants, *continued*

Problems That Interfere with Adequate Suck

Problem	Factors Which Cause or Exacerbate	Treatment Techniques
weak suck: results in inefficient feeding and generates inadequate pressure on the nipple	• overall weakness from medical compromise (premature infant) • respiratory problems • endurance problems	• Position child appropriately. • Use firm jaw and cheek support. • Use a small bottle. (This allows you to hold it and still provide the jaw and cheek stability.) • Gently try to pull the nipple from the child's mouth to promote stronger sucking. • Slightly increase the bolus size. (Note: If the bolus becomes too large, the child will cough and choke.) • Establish non-nutritive suck.
excessive jaw movement: may result in abnormal tongue movement and lip seal may be compromised	• jaw instability, which may be the result of inappropriate tone • premature infants have not developed tone in bulk in the oral-facial muscles • neck hyperextension may yield jaw instability • low oral-facial tone or facial weakness • abnormal tongue movements	• Make sure head and neck are aligned or with a slight flexion. • Provide some pressure with a finger under the child's jaw to help grade the movement of the jaw. (Make sure the pressure is on the mandible and not on the base of the tongue as this may interfere with sucking.) • Try bringing the child's head into more neck flexion with the chin closer to the chest. This way, the chest provides stability for the jaw. Carefully monitor the child's respiratory patterns.

continued

The Source for Pediatric Dysphagia

Chapter 6: Treatment Techniques for Infants, *continued*

Problem	Factors Which Cause or Exacerbate	Treatment Techniques
weak latch/open mouth; disinterested	• poor arousal • poor hunger signals • stress • low oral-motor tone • infant trying to maintain open airway	• Arouse the infant. • Use lingual stroking or tapping to increase tone and facilitate forward tongue position. • Apply firm pressure to palate. • If it's an airway problem, you may need to defer oral feeding. • Use organizing techniques.
poor lip seal: The negative pressure suction for sucking or suckling may be reduced if the seal on the nipple is broken. You will hear a smacking sound when suction is lost. You may also see loss of the formula from the corners of the mouth or lower lip.	• decreased muscle tone or weakness (e.g., prematurity) • Excessive jaw movements and wide jaw excursions make it difficult for the child to maintain lip closure. • Abnormal tongue movements with strong protrusion may push fluid out of the infant's mouth. • absent or small sucking pads	• Provide external support to cheeks and lips to help the child close her lips around the nipple. • Put your thumb and index finger (or middle finger) on the sucking pads to help the child purse her lips. • Child may need some jaw support. • Try using a smaller bottle. (This allows you to hold the bottle and still reach around it to provide jaw and lip-cheek support.)

continued

Chapter 6: Treatment Techniques for Infants, *continued*

Problem	Factors Which Cause or Exacerbate	Treatment Techniques
poor initiation of sucking: If a baby is hungry but cannot initiate sucking, he becomes even fussier.	• Child may have a hyperactive root reflex and will keep rooting for the nipple rather than latching on. • Infant has her mouth wide open and is unable to close her mouth to start sucking. • Infant may have ineffective tongue protrusion or a mildly hypersensitive response which prevents the beginning of sucking. • If the child is overly hungry, she may have problems initiating sucking.	• Provide control of the head through positioning to decrease excessive rooting. • Put the nipple on the midline of the baby's tongue, apply downward pressure, and provide cheek support. • If the child has trouble closing her mouth, assist with jaw control.
tremors	• stress • neurological deficits	• Use calming/organizing techniques.
munching	• disorganization • abnormal movement pattern • may be compensatory for poor latch	• Apply external support to jaw. • Use organizing techniques.
retracted and elevated tongue	• stress • poor arousal • compensation for lack of stability • neck is hyperextended	• Elicit non-nutritive suck. • Use lingual stroking/tapping. • Provide head/neck support by placing your hand behind the infant's head or holding the infant against your chest. (Note: Do not try to force nipple.)

continued

Chapter 6: Treatment Techniques for Infants, *continued*

Problem	Factors Which Cause or Exacerbate	Treatment Techniques
tongue bunching	• stress/refusal • disorganization • hypertonicity	• Use organizing techniques. • Give infant a break. • Establish non-nutritive suck. • Use lingual stroking/tapping.
low lingual cupping	• poor oral-motor tone (hypertonic or hypotonic) • excessive jaw excursions	• Use lingual stroking/tapping. • Provide external jaw support.
tongue protrusion	• stress/refusal • macroglossia • Down Syndrome • related to hypotonia • seen after lengthy intubation	• Give infant a break. • Establish non-nutritive suck. • Try larger, broader based nipple.

In Chapter 1, the importance of coordination between sucking, swallowing, and breathing was described. If the infant has timed and coordinated these three events, it should result in a very rhythmic pattern. Problems associated with the coordination of sucking, swallowing, and breathing are indicated in the chart on the next page (Wolf and Glass, 1992; Agnos, 1998).

Chapter 6: Treatment Techniques for Infants, *continued*

Problems Associated with Coordinating Sucking, Swallowing, and Breathing

Problem	Factors Which Cause or Exacerbate	Treatment Techniques
prolonged sucking (i.e., feeding-induced apnea): An infant may show long sucking bursts without breathing at appropriate intervals. The child may then experience what is described by Wolf and Glass (1992) as feeding-induced apnea. The child's oxygen levels drop (desaturate) and the child may experience bradycardia. Feeding-induced apnea may be more noted at the beginning of a feeding than toward the middle or end. Other characteristics include excessive spillage from mouth, audible gulping, or catch-up breathing. The pattern appears to be more common in premature babies.	prematurity (although it may occur in full-term babies)	• The feeder can provide the appropriate pacing for the baby. After 3-5 suck-swallows, remove the nipple from the child's mouth so the child can breathe. Keep the nipple in contact with the baby's lips so the baby knows you have not totally removed it. • Tilt the bottle downward to stop the flow of liquid. • Allow very young premature infants (32 to 35 weeks) to postpone nipple feeding until more mature. (You may need to wait only one week.) • Decrease the rate of flow to reduce the frequency of swallowing. This may allow the child to organize the suck-swallow-breathing pattern more readily. Use baby rice cereal to thicken the liquids or use a slower-flow nipple.

continued

Chapter 6: Treatment Techniques for Infants, *continued*

Problem	Factors Which Cause or Exacerbate	Treatment Techniques
short sucking bursts: The baby may take only 1-3 sucks before pausing for multiple breaths.	• swallowing or respiratory difficulties • delayed swallow (Short sucking bursts may be the infant's adaptive response to the faulty mechanism.)	• Treatment techniques should be based on videofluoroscopic evaluation of swallowing. • Give breaks. • Check pacing. • Try sidelying position. • Provide increased respiratory support (e.g., supplemental oxygen).
disorganized sucking: characterized by disorganized and uneven pattern; coughing and choking are typically noted	• general neurological disorganization • mild respiratory problems • nipple flow rate incompatible with infant suck	• Bundle the infant to decrease extraneous movement. • Reduce extraneous noise and light. • Use rocking or music to help with rhythm. • Use gentle pacing (i.e., Take the bottle away after one or two sucks and allow a long pause.). • Reduce the flow rate (e.g., different nipple, thicker liquids). • Gradually introduce liquid by dipping a pacifier or your little finger into the formula and putting it into the baby's mouth.
fatigue or lethargy during feeding: often a reflection of an infant having to work too hard to breathe and eat	• poor coordination of breathing and eating	• Provide smaller amounts by mouth and increase gavage feeding. • Provide non-nutritive suck/oral stimulation during gavage feeding. • Reduce distractions in environment.

The Source for Pediatric Dysphagia

Chapter 6: Treatment Techniques for Infants, *continued*

Disorders in the Pharyngeal Stage of Swallowing

(Note: Disorders in the pharyngeal stage are most accurately diagnosed using a videofluoroscopic evaluation of swallowing.)

Problem	Factors Which Cause or Exacerbate	Treatment Techniques
delayed swallow with aspiration before the swallow: The greater the delay triggering the pharyngeal swallow, the greater the risk of aspiration.	• neurological dysfunction	• It is almost impossible to provide thermal stimulation on an infant, so you might try very cold formula or thicker foods that are very cold. • The baby can suck a frozen pacifier. Fill the pacifier with water and then freeze. You may need several frozen pacifiers for one session. (To freeze a pacifier, drill a hole in the back side of the pacifier. Be sure not to drill through the nipple. Fill with water and freeze.) • Help the baby control the bolus. Allow the baby to get only one bolus and then swallow. A single bolus should be 0.1-0.5 cc in size. Use an open nipple and put in only that amount of fluid. • Wolf and Glass describe a method to control bolus sizes through a 20 cc feeding syringe attached to a 5 flange gavage feeding tube. (See page 121.) The feeding tube is taped to the nipple of the pacifier. As the baby sucks, small boluses of liquid can be released by squeezing the syringe into the baby's mouth at an appropriate rate.

continued

Chapter 6: Treatment Techniques for Infants, *continued*

Problem	Factors Which Cause or Exacerbate	Treatment Techniques
aspiration during the swallow: You may observe coughing.	• may be due to insufficient closure and elevation of the larynx	• Bring head forward into a significant chin tuck. • Use an angled-neck bottle to keep the child in neck flexion. • Thicken the feedings with rice cereal. • Slow flow rate (e.g., nipple with smaller hole, thicker feedings). • Re-alert infant.
aspiration after the swallow: may be due to residue in the pharynx. These infants may have wet and noisy breathing, especially after feeding.	• may be due to residue in the pharynx	• Modify the food consistency if the videofluoroscopic study shows that the child does better with certain consistencies. • Encourage multiple dry swallows by having the baby suck on a pacifier after a single bolus is presented. • Have the baby swallow thin liquid as a wash if this has been shown to be effective on videofluoroscopy.

Chapter 6: Treatment Techniques for Infants, continued

References

Agnos, S. "Pediatric Swallowing Disorders." TFG, Inc. Conference at Nashville, TN, 1998.

Arvedson, J. and Brodsky, L. *Pediatric Swallowing and Feeding: Assessment and Management*, San Diego: Singular Publishing Group, Inc., 1993, pp. 5-12.

Brazelton, T.B. *Neo-natal Behavioral Assessment Scale*, Philadelphia: J.D. Lippincott Company, 1984.

Comrie, J.D. and Helm, J.M. "Common Feeding Problems in the Intensive Care Nursery: Maturation, Organization, Evaluation, and Management Strategies." *Seminars in Speech and Language*, Vol. 18, No. 3, 1997, pp. 239-261.

Morris, S.E. and Klein, M.D. *Pre-Feeding Skills: A Comprehensive Resource for Feeding Development*, San Antonio: Therapy Skill Builders, a division of The Psychological Corporation, 1987.

Rosen, C.L. et al. "Hypoxemia Associated with Feeding in the Pre-term and Full-Term Neonate." *American Journal of Diseases in Children*, Vol. 138, 1984, pp. 623-628.

Rosenthal, S. et al. *Dysphagia and the Child with Developmental Disabilities: Medical, Clinical, and Family Interventions*, San Diego: Singular Publishing Group, Inc., 1995.

Selley, W.G. and Boxall, J. "A New Way to Treat Sucking and Swallowing Difficulties in Babies." *The Lancet*, 1991, pp. 1182-1184.

Tuchman, D. and Walter, R. *Disorders of Feeding and Swallowing in Infants and Children: Pathophysiology, Diagnosis, and Treatment*, San Diego: Singular Publishing Group, Inc., 1994.

White-Traut, R.C. and Hutchens, C.M. "Modulating Infant State in Premature Infants." *Journal of Pediatric Nursing*, Vol. 2, 1987, pp. 96-101.

Wolf, L.F. and Glass, R.P. *Feeding and Swallowing Disorders in Infancy: Assessment and Management*, San Antonio: Therapy Skill Builders, a division of The Psychological Corporation, 1992.

Chapter 7: Breast-feeding and the Child with a Feeding Disorder

Mothers of infants with disabilities and low birth weights have been discouraged from breast-feeding in the past due to possible inadequate nutritional content of the breast milk and/or feeding difficulties which require special assistance. It was also felt that breast-feeding was considered to be more work than bottle feeding. There was concern that an infant's physiological stability is compromised with the use of breast-feeding (Meyer and Brown, 1996). However, recent research indicates that early breast-feedings are less stressful physiologically than are early bottle feedings (Hill et al.,1997; Meyer and Brown, 1996). In fact, stimulation from breast-feeding and closeness to the mother can aid an infant's respiratory function (Rosenthal et al., 1993).

Breast-feeding should not be eliminated as an option if an infant has oral-motor difficulties because adaptations can be made. However, implementation of breast-feeding should be considered with an awareness of the possibility of starvation, specifically with a premature infant (Lawrence, 1989). Pre-term infants may have difficulty with breast-feeding until they are at a 37-week gestational age. Low birth weight infants initiate and continue with breast-feeding less frequently than do full term, healthy babies. In addition, few low birth weight babies are able to initiate breast-feeding resulting in mothers needing to express their milk (Young, 1993). Despite these concerns, mothers with children with disabilities should be encouraged to try breast-feeding as the advantages of breast-feeding as described below remain unchanged (Lotze, 1995).

Advantages and Disadvantages of Breast-feeding

The benefits of breast-feeding have been discussed for centuries. (See page 175.) In 1978, the American Academy of Pediatrics began to promote breast-feeding as the optimal source of nutrition for most infants younger than six months of age (Hill et al., 1997). Breast milk is the resource for nutrition and in many cases the most cost effective and convenient nutritional source (Young, 1993).

There are instances when breast-feeding should be avoided, such as when the mother's diet is inadequate, when substance abuse is suspected, or when the mother has been diagnosed with a disease that may be transmitted via the milk (e.g., HIV/AIDS, Herpes) (Pereira and Barbosa, 1986). However, it seems that the benefits of breast-feeding far exceed the disadvantages of breast feeding with low birth weight infants, pre-term infants, and children with disabilities (Meyer and Brown, 1986).

How Breast-feeding Works

Despite the many benefits of breast-feeding for infants, the process is not always an easy one. Milk is expressed quite differently from the breast than from a bottle. Wolf and Glass (1992) describe the importance of the infant's sucking performance in the initiation of the flow or "let-down" of milk. With breast-feeding, milk is ejected from the alveoli to the nipple as the pituitary gland

Chapter 7: Breast-feeding and the Child with a Feeding Disorder, continued

Advantages of Breast-feeding	Disadvantages of Breast-feeding
nutritionally superior to formula	difficult to measure intake
fewer allergic reactions	difficulty latching on
well tolerated	potentially slower with children with disabilities
convenient	influenced by mother's PO intake
cost effective	
facilitates good tongue and jaw development	
aids respiratory function	
fewer infections and/or protection from infection	
greater post-discharge weight gain	

releases a chemical substance. This "let-down" may occur several times during a feeding. However, the flow of milk does not continue without stimulation either from sucking, infant cries, or the mother thinking of the infant (Wolf and Glass, 1992).

The way milk is expressed from the breast was first reported by Ardran et al. in 1958 using cineradiographic imaging. The infant holds the nipple between his tongue and hard palate with his tongue tip at the gums. The synchronized movement of both the jaw and tongue elevating in conjunction with the rhythmical oral posterior tongue movement results in the expression of milk. Once the milk moves posteriorly, a voluntary swallow is initiated (Arvedson et al., 1993). More recent research by Smith et al. (1998) adds that the tongue cups around the nipple to assist with milk expression. Close lip approximation is needed for successful breast-feeding, however, failure to achieve close lip approximation does not preclude breast-feeding (Wolf and Glass, 1992).

The majority of milk is expressed from each breast within the first four minutes, although infants may continue to suck for pleasure purposes (Bosma, 1986). The suck/swallow sequence occurs in approximately one second, though sporadic interruptions may occur. It is when the interruptions become more frequent and/or affect the organization of the suck/swallow that one should be concerned. Infants may suck from each breast for equal amounts of time though

Chapter 7: Breast-feeding and the Child with a Feeding Disorder, continued

the volume is not correlated to the time spent on the breast. As a child develops, less time is spent on the breast. Intake remains unchanged due to increased skill of the infant as well as the mother's having a quicker "let-down" (Wolf and Glass, 1992).

Ardran et al. (1958) reported that the sucking pattern, including the jaw and tongue movement, occurs within one to five seconds while Wolf and Glass (1992) reported a high variability in sucking patterns. They report that the sucking rate increases at the start of feeding, decreases once the "let-down" occurs, and increases as the feeding continues. They explain this variability as being dependent on the volume of the flow of milk.

Readiness for Breast-feeding

Successful breast-feeding is not only dependent on the mechanics of sucking, but, according to Lothian (1995), also on the infant's behavior, including alertness, stamina, and ability to self-regulate. Alertness and stamina are important for breast-feeding because a child's failure to stay awake during the nursing process will affect her performance. An infant's failure to latch on for an adequate amount of time will inhibit the production or flow of milk which results in inadequate intake. Adequacy of intake and efficiency are imperative for all newborns, but are more important for children with special needs.

A child's ability to self-regulate, or independently calm and settle, is a contributing factor to the child's success with breast-feeding. A child who is difficult to soothe may have more difficulty with breast-feeding as the mother's confidence and satisfaction are diminished. As stated previously, the mother's emotional status may interfere with breast-feeding success. However, other contributing factors are the ability of the mother to recognize the child's difficulty or inefficiency and then compensate for the child's difficulty.

Wolf and Glass (1992) have described four factors which must be in place for successful breast-feeding.

1. The anatomical structure of the breast and nipple must be adequate to provide a storage system and exit channels.
2. The secretion of milk must be initiated and maintained.
3. Milk must be ejected or propelled from the areola to the nipple.
4. The baby must be able to receive the milk and provide ongoing stimuli for further secretion and ejection of milk.

Problems That Can Occur with Breast-feeding

Breast-feeding problems include breast pain or infection, inadequate milk supply, inadequate diet of the mother, inappropriate handling of the infant, irregular feeding schedules, and unpredictable emotional state. Lawrence (1989) provides a flowchart for failure to thrive while breast-feeding which summarizes problems that may be encountered. (See page 177.)

Chapter 7: Breast-feeding and the Child with a Feeding Disorder, continued

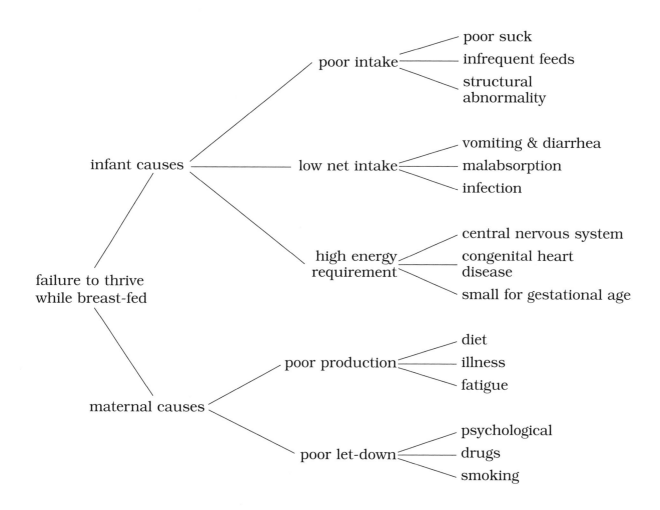

Diagnostic flowchart for failure to thrive. Reprinted with permission from R.A. Lawrence, *Breast-feeding: A Guide for the Medical Profession*, St. Louis: C.V. Mosby Co., 1989.

If the problems are related to the mother, they may be handled by a breast-feeding specialist called a lactation nurse or lactation specialist. However, oral-motor feeding problems may also be the cause for the difficulty a mother and child are having with feeding. If that is the case, the SLP should be involved in the evaluation and treatment. Whenever an infant/mother pair are having difficulties with breast-feeding, consider both the mother and the infant and the relationship between the physical and emotional status of both. When a child has difficulty with sucking, the mother may become emotionally stressed, and therefore have a decreased milk supply. Contributing to this situation may be the infant becoming more hungry and showing irritability and lack of interest. These factors will only lead to more frustration on the mother's part (Wolf and Glass, 1992). The La Leche League can also be a resource for mothers who are breast-feeding children with feeding problems.

Chapter 7: Breast-feeding and the Child with a Feeding Disorder, continued

Sucking problems may occur due to structural problems, temperament, or endurance. The infant's failure to adequately compress the nipple and hold it securely will result in insufficient ability to trigger the "let-down" reflex. The infant's inability to compress and sustain the compression as well as demonstrate rhythmical tongue movement may result in an inadequate milk expression. Failure to express milk efficiently will result in fatigue prior to the attainment of adequate nutrition (Morris and Klein, 1987). Oral hypersensitivity in conjunction with a tonic bite reflex can lead to the mother's discomfort.

Suggestions for Intervention

Strong Tongue Tip-to-Alveolar Ridge Contact — When an infant demonstrates strong tongue tip-to-alveolar ridge (palate) contact, it is difficult to place the breast nipple in the child's mouth. Due to soft breast tissue, it is difficult to provide adequate resistance to encourage the child's tongue to lower to allow the nipple to enter the mouth. Encouraging a wide mouth opening to break the tongue tip-to-alveolar ridge/palate contact may facilitate nipple placement. Postural change is needed if extensive tongue tip elevation is used as a means to stabilize (e.g., hypotonic babies). Postural changes include positions that prompt neck elongation and forward head flexion. Quick swiping or vibration and downward pressure to the tongue tip may also help bring the tongue tip down (Wolf and Glass, 1992).

Tongue Retraction — When tongue retraction is present, contact between the nipple and the tongue is limited. Without this contact, the infant may be unable to achieve pressure against the nipple, thus not allowing milk to be expressed. The use of a nipple shield may be indicated as it will help elongate the nipple and allow for tongue/nipple contact. A nipple shield is a silicone/latex device shaped like a sombrero that fits over the nipple. Nipple shields should be used cautiously, specifically with infants with limited strength, as milk flow is restricted. Providing firm downward pressure to the infant's tongue before or during feeding may also be beneficial (Wolf and Glass 1992).

Poor Central Grooving — The inability to cup the nipple with the tongue makes expression difficult. A child may attempt to compensate for this failure by demonstrating tongue protrusion and nipple "chewing." Midline tongue pressure may encourage tongue cupping along with the use of lingual stroking or tapping and external jaw support. However, if these strategies are not effective, the nipple shield may be beneficial (Wolf and Glass, 1992).

The Source for Pediatric Dysphagia

Chapter 7: Breast-feeding and the Child with a Feeding Disorder, *continued*

Hypotonia An infant with hypotonia may have a weak suck which results in the inadequate expression of milk and possibly inadequate nutrition. However, in conjunction with the use of vibration, firm pressure, and proper positioning, breast feeding is possible (Rosenthal et al., 1993).

Hypertonia Hypertonia may result in an arching behavior, making it difficult for the mother to maintain positioning necessary for breast-feeding (Rosenthal et al., 1993). Measures should be taken to ensure proper positioning to facilitate feeding. In addition, the infant may have increased tone in the face. Application of firm pressure along the sides of the infant's nose and mouth and vibration to the cheeks and lips may be used to help reduce tone in these oral-facial structures.

Recessed Jaw When a smaller recessed jaw is present, the tongue may not move forward and compress the nipple as is needed for milk expression. The strategies used with tongue tip elevation, tongue retraction, and poor central grooving of the tongue may be helpful. In addition, forward pressure to the lower jaw may be helpful in assisting with compression (Wolf and Glass, 1992).

Short Frenulum Inability to extend the tongue may result in an incomplete seal between the tongue and the nipple. Ankyloglossia may cause the child to have difficulty latching on which can cause sore nipples or poor weight gain. The severity of anklyloglossia varies as do the complications. A short frenulum may be clipped surgically if it interferes with breast-feeding (Berg, 1990; Wiessinger and Miller, 1995; Maimet et al., 1990). Currently, there are no guidelines relative to the severity or anatomical measurement of ankyloglossia which conclusively indicates the need for a frenulectomy. It is through the evaluation of the infant's oral-motor function and the mother's nipple that a problem is determined.

Excessive Jaw Excursion With excessive jaw excursion, an infant may have difficulty obtaining and maintaining compression of the nipple between the tongue and hard palate. Strategies to assist include postural changes (e.g., head and neck support to eliminate the infant pushing away or pulling away from the breast). Jaw and cheek stability may also be helpful and can be provided by the mother during breast-feeding (Wolf and Glass, 1992; Morris and Klein, 1987).

Chapter 7: Breast-feeding and the Child with a Feeding Disorder, continued

Inadequate Mouth Opening	Failure of the child to open his mouth for the breast can be facilitated by using arousal techniques such as gentle, firm, unpredictable movements; bouncing while supporting the head and neck; rocking from side to side, pressure to the jaw to open the mouth; and vibration to the mouth. Auditory techniques include talking to the baby while varying pitch and loudness or by playing loud music.
Mouth/Breast Mismatch	In conjunction with assessing a child's oral-motor function, it is also imperative that the mother's nipples be assessed to determine compliance between the oral-motor abilities and the mother's nipple characteristics. For example, a child with a retracted tongue or strong tongue tip to alveolar ridge contact may have difficulty with the mother's nipple if it is a short nipple or if it is not as rigid as a bottle nipple (Wolf and Glass, 1992).
Behavior and State	The infant's ability to arouse and maintain arousal are key to successful breast-feeding. Providing the appropriate stimulation and techniques to modify and enhance the behavior are dependent on the child's state (Wolf and Glass, 1992). Treatment techniques were reviewed in Chapter 6 and they include movement, auditory, and tactile stimulation.

Transition from Tube Feeding

Children who initially are fed via tubes are able to transition to breast-feeding, though the success of this transition is dependent on the specific problems the child is having, the age of the infant, and the occurrence of a tonic bite reflex. When a mother has a desire to breast-feed, she may be able to do so with assistance and encouragement. Oral sensory stimulation may be needed (Morris and Klein, 1987). Wolf and Glass (1992) state that three ideas should be kept in mind when considering breast-feeding after tube feeding:

- adequacy of PO intake and growth and development

- adequacy of breast milk expression

- maintenance of a milk supply

A Final Note About Breast-feeding

Breast-feeding is an enjoyable process and has been proven to be beneficial to both the mother and the child. However, breast-feeding is not for everyone, nor is it a successful event for all who attempt it. Mothers should be aware that breast-feeding can be difficult for even the full-term healthy baby, and that it is not a natural process for all infants.

Chapter 7: Breast-feeding and the Child with a Feeding Disorder, *continued*

This does not mean that mothers should be discouraged if they desire to breast-feed. Breast-feeding alone may not be the best practice for adequate nutrition, but providing the mother with the option of combining breast-feeding with bottle feeding or a supplemental nursing system should be presented. Most importantly, educate the mother and be a resource for her.

Chapter 7: Breast-feeding and the Child with a Feeding Disorder, *continued*

References

Ardran, G.M. et al. "A Cineradiographic Study of Breast-feeding." *British Journal of Radiology*, Vol. 31, 1958, pp. 156-162.

Arvedson, J. et al. "Anatomy, Embryology, and Physiology." In Arvedson, J.C. and Brodsky, L. (eds.) *Pediatric Swallowing and Feeding: Assessment and Management*, San Diego: Singular Publishing Group, Inc., 1993, pp. 44-45.

Berg, K.L. "Tongue-Tie (Ankyloglossia) and Breast-feeding: A Review." *Journal of Human Lactation*, Vol. 6, No. 3, 1990, pp. 109-112.

Hill P.D. et al. "Breast-feeding of Low Birth Weight Infants after Hospital Discharge." *Journal of Obstetrics, Gynecological, and Neonatal Nursing*, Vol. 26, No. 2, 1997, pp. 189-198.

Lawrence, R. *Breast-feeding: A Guide for the Medical Profession*, 3rd ed., Boston: Jones and Bartlett, 1989.

Lothian, J.A. "It Takes Two to Breast-feed: The Baby's Role in Successful Breast-feeding." *Journal of Nurse/Midwifery*, Vol. 40, No. 4, 1995, pp. 328-334.

Lotze, M. "Nursing Assessment and Management." In Rosenthal, S.R. et al. (eds.) *Dysphagia and the Child with Developmental Disabilities: Medical, Clinical and Family Interventions*, San Diego: Singular Publishing Group, Inc., 1995, pp. 333-339.

Maimet, C. et al. "Neonatal Frenotomy May Be Necessary to Correct Breast-feeding Problems." *Journal of Human Lactation*, Vol. 6, No. 7, 1990, pp. 117-121.

McBride, M.C. and Danner, S.C. "Sucking Disorders in Neurologically Impaired Infants: Assessment and Facilitation of Breast-feeding." *Clinics in Perinatology*, Vol. 14, No.1, 1987, pp. 109-131.

Medoff-Cooper, B. "Changes in Nutritive Sucking Patterns with Increasing Gestational Age." *Nursing Research*, Vol. 40, No. 4, 1991, pp. 245-247.

Medoff-Cooper, B. and Ray, W. "Neonatal Sucking Behavior." *Image: Journal of Nursing Scholarships*, Vol. 27, 1995, pp. 195-199.

Meier, T.P. et al. "Breast-feeding Support Services in the Neonatal Intensive-Care Unit." *Journal of Obstetrics, Gynecological, and Neonatal Nursing-Clinical Studies*, Vol. 31, 1992, pp. 338-347.

Meier, T.P. and Brown, L.P. "State of the Science: Breast-feeding for Mothers and Low Birth Weight Infants." *Nursing Clinics of North America*, Vol. 31, No. 2, 1996, pp. 351-365.

Morris, S.E. and Klein, D. *Pre-Feeding Skills: A Comprehensive Resource for Feeding Development*, San Antonio: Therapy Skill Builders, a division of The Psychological Corporation, 1987.

Chapter 7: Breast-feeding and the Child with a Feeding Disorder, *continued*

Pereira, G.R. and Barbosa, N.M.M. "Controversies in Neonatal Nutrition." *Pediatric Clinics of North America*, Vol. 33, No. 1, 1986, pp. 65-89.

Smith, W.L. et al. "Imaging Evaluation of the Human Nipple during Breast-feeding." *American Journal of Diseases of Children*, Vol. 142, 1988, pp. 76-78.

Steichen, J. et al. "Breast-feeding the Low Birth Weight Pre-term Infant." *Clinics in Perinatology*, Vol. 14, 1987, pp. 131-171.

Weissinger, D. and Miller, M. "Breast-feeding Difficulties as a Result of a Tight Lingual and Labial Frena: A Case Report." *Journal of Human Lactation*, Vol. 11, No. 4, 1995, pp. 313-316.

Wolf, L.F. and Glass, R.P. *Feeding and Swallowing Disorders in Infancy: Assessment and Management*, San Antonio: Therapy Skill Builders, a division of The Psychological Corporation, 1992.

Chapter 8: Behavioral Feeding Problems

Behavioral feeding problems are those that have components of both motivational problems (i.e., choice) and skill deficits (i.e., lack of ability) (Babbitt et al., 1994). What starts as a physiologically-based problem may become a behavioral problem, often making it difficult to differentiate the two. Problems can be as severe as needing supplemental tube feedings or as mild as a child whose caloric intake is inadequate because of excessive juice consumption (Smith and Lifshitz, 1994).

With the exception of colic, early feeding difficulties may have a significant impact on growth. Growth can continue to be affected as long as the feeding problems persist (Dahl and Kristiansson, 1987). Various terms used to describe children with behavioral feeding problems include non-organic failure to thrive (Bithoney and Rathburn, 1983), growth failure secondary to feeding skill disorders (Ramsey et al., 1993), functional dysphagia (Carstens, 1982), conversion dysphagia (Kanner, 1935 in Atkins et al., 1994), and conditioned dysphagia (Di Scipio et al., 1978).

Children may present with a purely behavioral feeding disorder, or there may be a behavioral component to a physiological problem (e.g., cleft palate, cerebral palsy). At the conclusion of the feeding assessment, it is important to differentiate which components of a feeding disorder are behavioral in nature and then to establish goals accordingly.

A feeding problem may be behavioral if:

- Child fails to achieve expected weight/height thresholds.
- Parents report that feeding is a "battle."
- Parents report excessively long mealtimes.
- Child snacks frequently on junk food, but will not eat a "real meal."
- Child frequently gags or vomits during a meal.
- Child is highly selective about food.
- Child simply refuses food.
- Child holds food in her mouth.

Causes of Behavioral Feeding Problems

There may be a single cause or there may be a combination of causes resulting in a behavioral feeding problem.

1. Medical problems that lead to delay in initiating food by mouth. The reason for the initial problem may no longer exist, but the child may remain reluctant/unable to take food orally (e.g., A child may have had a TE fistula preventing oral feeding. The fistula may be repaired, but feeding problems persist.).

2. The child has passed the critical period for the introduction of food (Illingsworth and Lister, 1964). If children are not given solid food to chew at the time when they are first able to chew (around 6 months), problems

Chapter 8: Behavioral Feeding Problems, *continued*

with eating solids are more likely to occur later. The age of readiness differs from child to child and may in fact be missed in some children, particularly those with delays, if the child's development is not monitored closely.

3. Children with neurological disorders may present with respiratory difficulties as a result of poor coordination of sucking/swallowing with breathing. They may also exhibit hyperextension of the neck with scapular adduction and shoulder girdle elevation making swallowing difficult (Morris and Klein, 1987). Some children may not have a diagnosed neurological disorder, but may present with histories that indicate some form of neurological involvement and problems that manifest as different degrees of oral, sensorimotor, and pharyngeal dysphagia (Ramsay et al., 1993).

4. Recurrent trauma such as NG placement, suctioning, or other invasive procedures during infancy may make the child fearful of being touched on the face and/or mouth (Di Scipio, 1978).

5. Psychosocial factors (e.g., forced feeding, sexual abuse, negative eating associations, family eating and mealtime routines, dysfunctional family, maternal inadequacies) (Culbert, 1996)

6. Psychiatric disorder (e.g., an anxiety disorder or depression) (Atkins, 1994)

Certain groups of children, such as those with developmental disabilities and those with mental retardation, run a high risk for feeding problems that may have some behavioral feeding component. The following factors also increase the risk of feeding problems (Singer, 1990):

- Congenital Heart Disease
- Cystic Fibrosis
- Phenylketonuria and other metabolic disorders
- Cancer
- Diabetes Mellitus
- Asthma
- Gastrointestinal Disorders
    - Inflammatory bowel disease
    - Esophagitis
    - Acute gastroenteritis
    - Irritable bowel syndrome
    - Encopresis
    - Gastroesophageal reflux
- Bronchopulmonary Dysplasia
- Cerebral Palsy
- Gastrostomy
- History of tube feeding
- Cleft lip and palate
- Down Syndrome
- Autism
- Spina Bifida
- Myelodysplasia

The Source for Pediatric Dysphagia

Chapter 8: Behavioral Feeding Problems, continued

In addition, Singer lists the following as predisposing factors for feeding problems: hyperactive gag reflex, long-term tube or intravenous drip feedings, larger than normal caloric requirements, difficult temperament, decreased social responsivity, prematurity, and low birth weight.

Education to Prevent Problems

Parental education is necessary to prevent/reduce problems in children whose medical diagnosis increases the risk of feeding problems (e.g., developmental disorders, esophageal problems) and for children presenting with very mild problems which may get worse if not addressed early. Parents need to have knowledge of normal development of feeding transitions and guidelines for early feeding experiences. See Appendix 8-A (pages 208-209) for a parental handout on ways to minimize behavioral feeding problems and ways to take the stress out of mealtimes.

Assessment

A disorder needs to be addressed when parents voice a concern that their child is exhibiting a problem, when the child is judged as underweight (without a physiological reason), or when termination of tube feeding does not result in the child taking anticipated amount/variety of food/liquid. Assessment needs to be multi-disciplinary even if a structured "feeding team" is not available. Besides the SLP, each of the following can play a key role: pediatrician, dietitian, occupational therapist, behavioral psychologist, and social worker.

Components of the Evaluation

A medical assessment should include a modified barium swallow to rule out aspiration or other pharyngeal dysphagia problems. It should also include gastrointestinal studies to rule out esophageal dismotility, gastroesophageal reflux, and gastric emptying problems.

A physical examination is needed to assess status on growth charts to indicate current weight/height adequacy and to rule out neurological involvement. Ramsay et al. (1993) state that in a group of children with non-organic failure to thrive, half of them had histories that indicated neurological involvement even though they had no diagnosed neurological disorder. Presence or absence of food allergies also needs to be determined.

An assessment of family issues should determine caregiver psychological variables (e.g., marital conflict, neglect, depression, family dynamics); caregiver social variables (e.g., poverty, lack of nutritional information, improper feeding techniques) (Lachenmeyer, 1995); and financial and educational resources.

Chapter 8: Behavioral Feeding Problems, continued

Prior to the initial feeding evaluation, ask the primary caregiver to complete a *Food Diary* for one week. (See pages 204-205.) The food diary should include:

- time of meals
- duration of meals
- location of meals
- location of child (e.g., high chair, floor, etc.)
- people present
- if child is fed, who did the feeding
- type of food eaten and/or presented
- amount taken at each meal
- child's behavior in response to the food
- caregiver's response to "problem" behaviors

It is also important to complete a case history form. (See Chapter 3, pages 86-87 and 109-112).

The Feeding Evaluation

Ask the caregiver to bring food and feeding utensils from home to make the feeding evaluation as much like the "usual" feeding patterns as possible. It will also be necessary to have a variety of other foods available to further assess preferences for flavors, texture, and temperature. (See page 64.) Although parents can provide significant information on food preferences, it has been reported that they are not always completely accurate (Parsons and Reid, 1990).

The seating arrangement should be as close as possible to what the child is used to. The caregiver should feed the child or allow the child to eat, depending on what usually happens. Observe and assess the following areas, as applicable. You can use the 4-month and older feeding evaluation (Chapter 3, pages 102-104) and the supplemental *Observation of Eating* Form. (See pages 206-207.)

1. Ability to maintain sitting for sufficient amount of time
2. Ability to self feed
3. Ability to handle various textures, flavors, and temperatures
4. Overall reaction to food (e.g., anticipation, interest, disinterest, anger, frustration, fear, crying, gagging, vomiting)
5. Oral-motor skill assessment to include sensitivity, chew, bite, suck, tongue movement, jaw control, and ability to clear bolus after swallow
6. Child's response to caregiver
7. Caregiver's response to child

Careful analysis of the information obtained on the evaluation and supplemental observation form should allow you to determine if the child is presenting with a behavioral feeding disorder, a physiological feeding disorder, or a combination of both. Determine the severity of the disorder. Behavioral feeding problems can be

Chapter 8: Behavioral Feeding Problems, continued

mild (e.g., the child fills up on juice instead of food) or severe (e.g., the child takes so little food that supplemental tube feeding is necessary).

Establishing a Plan of Treatment

After analyzing the type and severity of the feeding disorder, a treatment plan must be established. Careful consideration must be given to each of the following components.

1. Nutritional status: Will the child be able to maintain adequate nutrition/hydration on a full PO diet? Consult with the dietitian to help make this determination.

2. Behavioral vs. physiological components: Does the child have underlying physiological deficits that need to be addressed before the behavioral component can be addressed? Can any underlying physiological deficits be addressed at the same time a behavioral approach is initiated?

3. Caregiver variables: Determine the caregivers' perceptions of the problem. Do they understand how much of the problem is physiological vs. behavioral? What is the educational level of the caregivers? (This will affect how teaching occurs.) What are the caregivers' abilities to facilitate the treatment plan at home?

Antecedents and Consequences

It is also necessary to identify the relationship between antecedents (i.e., what happens immediately before) and consequences of (i.e., what happens immediately after) a behavior. By identifying and manipulating the variables that maintain a behavior, it then becomes easier to break the cycle of the behavior (Babbitt et al., 1994; Palmer et al., 1975).

Goals of Caregiver and Clinician

It is important to determine both the clinician's and the caregivers' goals. If there is not a good match between the caregivers' goals and the treatment plan established, there is little chance the goals will be met. By working together, a treatment plan can be established that is acceptable and workable.

Behavioral-Based Intervention

Behavioral intervention involves the use of a variety of behavioral techniques to change behavior (either increasing or decreasing it). Babbitt et al. (1994) describe behavioral feeding problems in terms of motivational disorders. Inappropriate behaviors (e.g., food refusal) are maintained by faulty reinforcement practices and skill deficits (e.g., inability to self-feed) remain due to lack of experience with a task.

Chapter 8: Behavioral Feeding Problems, *continued*

Before increasing, decreasing, changing, or teaching a behavior, the behavior itself must be operationally defined. Operationally defining a behavior means breaking the behavior down into component parts which can be learned and reinforced more easily than the whole behavior. For example, self feeding Cheerios® in milk could be operationally defined in the following way:

1. Child picks up the spoon.
2. Child moves the spoon toward the bowl with the cupped portion facing the bowl.
3. Child places the spoon in the cereal.
4. Child lifts the spoon out of the bowl maintaining its stability so that the Cheerios® stay on.
5. Child brings spoon toward mouth.
6. Child opens mouth.
7. Child closes mouth around the spoon.
8. Child removes the empty spoon from her mouth.
9. Child places spoon back in the bowl.

Breaking the activity down into smaller steps not only makes it easier to learn the activity, it also allows the feeding specialist to assess where the breakdown in performance lies and to place emphasis on that deficit.

In addition to breaking the activity into smaller steps, some clinicians begin to establish appropriate behavioral responses with non-feeding activities. Payne and Sheppard (1998) begin feeding therapy without introducing any food. They first teach the child to sit in the chair for very short periods of time, gradually increasing the length of time the child has to remain in the chair. They use several reinforcement techniques (e.g., positive reinforcement, negative reinforcement, extinction, etc.). After the child will sit for one minute, other non-feeding activities are introduced (e.g., child matches pictures or points to pictures on command). It is important that the task be a simple one that you know the child can complete.

Payne and Sheppard state that this teaches the child several lessons:

- You won't give the child anything to do that she cannot handle.

- You are the boss and are in control (since children with behavioral feeding problems often control the situation through their behavior).

- The child will be reinforced once the task is complete.

After the child complies on a variety of tasks, Payne and Sheppard begin to introduce food following the same principles.

Chapter 8: Behavioral Feeding Problems, *continued*

Techniques to Increase Behavior

Positive and negative reinforcement serve to increase the likelihood of a particular behavior.

Positive Reinforcement

Positive reinforcement involves adding something to the child's environment that was not present before. This increases the likelihood of that behavior happening again. Babbitt et al. (1994) provide the following example:

> A child takes a bite of food (behavior). The pleasant flavor of the food (which was previously absent) is sensed (consequence added), so using that set of circumstances (food is present but not in the mouth) the child is more likely to open his mouth for more (reinforcement).

Madsen and Thompson (1974) found that giving a child preferred foods (e.g., sugar-coated cereal) contingent on eating non-preferred foods was an effective reinforcement and therefore a means of increasing intake in normal preschoolers. Eating the non-preferred food was the behavior with the preferred foods as the consequence.

Similar findings were indicated in a study involving two children aged 6 and 9 (Riordan et al., 1980). Both had been admitted to a hospital that provided short-term interdisciplinary treatment for children and adolescents. One child was admitted for genetic screening and evaluation of retarded physical growth; the other was on her fourth admission due to weight loss and need for physical therapy. Before participating in treatment, both children had highly selective and inadequate diets. After reinforcement in which access to preferred foods was made contingent on accepting and then swallowing a non-preferred food, the children increased their consumption rate of selected foods, increased total number of grams per meal, and ate a more well-balanced diet.

Negative Reinforcement

Negative reinforcement gets a child out of a negative situation. It involves taking away something that is negative for the child that leads to the avoidance or an escape from a situation or stimulus (Babbitt et al., 1994). For example, if a child swallowed a predetermined amount of food, negative reinforcement would mean that the child would then be allowed to leave the table. Since the child does not want to be at the table, being allowed to leave after taking a bite is a negative reinforcement. Because the child was reinforced,

Chapter 8: Behavioral Feeding Problems, *continued*

she is more likely to eat the predetermined amount of food again the next time.

Negative and positive reinforcement can be used simultaneously. In the first example, each bite of the predetermined amount could be positively reinforced (e.g., verbal praise, "You did a great job eating that piece of apple!"), increasing the likelihood that the behavior would happen again. When the child has eaten the predetermined amount, negative reinforcement allows her to get down from the table.

Frequency of Reinforcement

It is necessary to gradually decrease the frequency of reinforcement so a specific behavior is maintained once reinforcement stops. For example, if the child was given verbal praise each time she took a bite of food, gradual cessation of reinforcement might mean that praise was given every 3 bites, then every 5 bites, then every 10 bites, and then only once or twice throughout the whole meal. Abrupt cessation of reinforcement may lead to an equally abrupt cessation of the target behavior. Changing the reinforcement schedule will be very child specific, so a thorough knowledge of what works for a child will be needed.

Techniques to Decrease Behavior

Positive and negative reinforcement increase target behaviors. Extinction, differential reinforcement of other behavior, antecedent manipulation, and punishment reduce or eliminate inappropriate behaviors (e.g., pushing food out of the mouth, refusing to open the mouth, yelling, and screaming) that interfere with appropriate feeding.

Extinction   Extinction is the termination of ongoing reinforcement. Extinction initially causes an increase in a behavior, but then leads to a decrease and possible elimination of a behavior. Babbitt et al. (1994) provide the example of a child who exhibits expulsion of food from his mouth which is negatively reinforced as the parents terminate the meal and let the child get down from the table. Extinction would involve continuing the meal and representing bites that have been expelled. Initially this will probably increase the frequency of expulsion, but it will eventually decrease the frequency leading to possible elimination of the behavior.

Time-out is another form of extinction whereby a child is removed from a reinforcing situation after exhibiting an inappropriate behavior. For example, a child who repeatedly refuses to eat an item might be told to get down from the table and stand with his back to the feeding therapist for a count of 10 or 20. This would be an effective time-out for a

Chapter 8: Behavioral Feeding Problems, continued

child who likes the interaction and loses the social contact with the adult. It is important to use time-out judiciously as time-out from an unpleasant situation (eating) can increase the likelihood that the inappropriate behavior will occur again to avoid the unpleasant situation.

Differential Reinforcement of Other Behavior

This involves getting rid of an unwanted behavior and replacing it with an acceptable one. It involves a combination of extinction (i.e., get rid of an unwanted behavior) and positive reinforcement (i.e., increase the likelihood of acceptable behavior). For example, a child throws a tantrum any time food other than a peanut butter and jelly sandwich is placed on her plate. As a consequence, she is allowed to leave the table (negative reinforcement of an unacceptable behavior). This negative reinforcement will most likely cause the tantrums to continue. If, however, the tantrum is ignored (extinction), and the child remains at the table and is given much praise (positive reinforcement) for at least trying and then eating what is on her plate, we are on the way to getting rid of the unacceptable behavior (tantrum) and promoting a desired behavior (eating a new food).

Antecedent Manipulation

This involves changing the course of events immediately prior to an unwanted behavior to decrease the likelihood that the behavior will occur. For example, if an unwanted behavior (tantrum) occurs because of the large amount of food on a child's plate, reducing the amount of food on the plate (antecedent manipulation) and then providing reinforcement to the child for eating all the food on her plate may reduce the possibility of a tantrum. The amount of food can be gradually increased.

Punishment

Punishment is the opposite of reinforcement. In reinforcement (positive or negative), a behavior occurs and is then reinforced which makes it more likely that the behavior will occur again. In punishment, a consequence is provided after a behavior. The consequence is intended to decrease the likelihood that that behavior will occur again. Babbitt et al. (1994) report that most punishment reported in feeding literature focuses on ruminative vomiting. Luiselli et al. (1993) used a combination of dietary manipulations, a pharmacological regimen, and behavioral strategies including use of verbal reprimand (punishment) to progressively reduce the frequency of ruminative vomiting. (See additional information on ruminative vomiting on pages 196-197.)

Chapter 8: Behavioral Feeding Problems, continued

Skill Acquisition Techniques

Skill Acquisition Techniques are designed to help children learn specific behaviors needed to be successful eaters which they have not learned due to lack of experience (e.g., A child who is NPO will not have had an opportunity to experience how to hold a spoon or handle a variety of consistencies.).

Prompting Prompting involves giving instruction and physical assistance to achieve a target behavior that has not been learned. For example, if the target behavior is getting food in the mouth via a spoon, instructions to the child may be, "Hold the spoon, open your mouth, and put the spoon in your mouth." Physical prompting may include your hand over the child's to pick up the spoon, placing the spoon in the bowl to collect the food, and then lifting the spoon toward the child's mouth.

Modeling Modeling describes the child's ability to master a task based on imitation of another, whether it's the feeding specialist, a parent, or a peer. Parents and peers can improve food preferences and eating habits by modeling eating a well-balanced diet (Finney, 1986) and observing more structured mealtimes (e.g., sitting at the table, TV off, etc.). Modeling can be an important part of generalization of behaviors outside treatment, as long as the behaviors modeled are appropriate.

Shaping a behavior Shaping involves gradually increasing the level of difficulty of a stimulus to achieve a higher level of complexity. Walco (1986) writes of the shaping involved to encourage a 13-year-old child to take pills. The child had a diagnosis of lymphocytic leukemia which required him to take a variety of pills. The problem was solved in two days using graded pieces of ice. Ice was chosen because it melts quickly and because the fear of it becoming lodged in the throat or causing gagging was felt to be minimal. It was felt that intrinsic motivation and the child's sense of accomplishment were adequate to maintain and generalize the behavior.

Generalization of Behavior

The ultimate goal of any feeding therapy program is for the child to use newly-learned behaviors in any setting with any person. Unless generalization is planned and executed as a component part of the treatment program, behaviors that are exhibited within the therapeutic environment may never be seen outside, thus reducing the efficacy of the program. When behaviors are stable within the treatment setting, new elements (e.g., people, places, foods, distractions, etc.) can be introduced in a systematic way (Babbitt et al., 1994).

Chapter 8: Behavioral Feeding Problems, *continued*

Other Therapeutic Approaches

Hypnobehavioral This approach has been found to be very successful with children who have choked or have a fear of choking on something (Culbert et al., 1996). These authors describe the study of a 6-year-old child who choked on a piece of hot dog. A physician who happened to be present saved the child with the Heimlich maneuver. Four days after this episode, the child became fearful of eating solid food for fear of choking. When the child was seen two weeks later for a feeding intervention, he was taking liquids only. Intervention took two visits and included using hypnotic language, imagery, and metaphors to allow the child to overcome the fear of eating. Such therapy would need to be carried out by a qualified behavioral psychologist.

Cognitive Behavioral This approach is reported to be particularly helpful with children who are experiencing food phobias. Carstens (1982) reported a case of a 12-year-old child who choked on a piece of pizza. Use of the Heimlich maneuver removed the pizza. In the days after the episode, the child avoided solid foods and then went to the emergency room reporting the sensation of something being "stuck" in his throat.

The boy was seen for one 90-minute treatment session. During the session, he was taught how to relax while eating, take deep breaths before or during a meal if he felt tension, chew each bite 20 times, take 10 swallows of water if the feeling of being "stuck" arose, and to seek out and correctly eat previously eaten foods. In addition, he was to serve himself a full meal three times each day and finish the entire helping of food and eat no sweets until the meal had been completed. This protocol worked very successfully, with the boy eating at will within a few days.

The hypothesis was that re-education in correct chewing and swallowing, combined with overcorrection using relaxation and swallowing resolved the problem. Carstens points out that the rapidity of treatment may be unusual and speculates that perhaps all that was needed in this case was the strong suggestion that relaxation and correct swallowing would solve the problem, in which case the treatment was a very effective placebo.

Pharmacological Arvedson (1997) reports that although pharmacological treatment and cognitive behavioral therapy is common in adults, it has not been used extensively with children. Atkins (1994) used alprazolam (i.e., Xanax®), a drug for anxiety

The Source for Pediatric Dysphagia

Chapter 8: Behavioral Feeding Problems, continued

disorders, with a 7-year-old child admitted to an in-patient psychiatric hospital following refusal of food after having choked on a piece of ham. In this case, there were multiple dysfunctional family issues, including a father who was allegedly physically and sexually abusive and alcohol dependent. During the hospital admission, the patient made insignificant progress with a behavioral reinforcement program, play therapy, and the allowance for the development of physiological hunger. The issue of fear of choking was judged to be the cause of the general lack of progress. At that point, alprazolam was prescribed. Once the dose reached 0.75 mg one hour before meals, the patient spontaneously reported decreased fear of choking and began to eat more. At discharge, he was eating normally after a gradual increase in texture from soft to firm.

Transactional Approach Arvedson (1997) states that this approach takes into consideration the combination of organic, psychological, and environmental factors. It involves the participation of various disciplines to create a comprehensive plan after discharge to include coping strategies for families, community resources to build a "team atmosphere" to convey trust, and support for the families.

Other Considerations

Forced Feeding Forced feeding is not an appropriate technique. It does not remediate the feeding problem because it does not promote voluntary consumption (Riordan et al., 1980). It may lead to the development of aspiration pneumonia (Davis in Perske et al., 1977) and may not be popular with parents which leads to parental noncompliance.

Justification for a modified method of forced feeding (Iwata et al., 1982) has included maximizing infrequent food acceptance with a positive reinforcement contingency and removing escape or avoidance. It involves providing physical prompts (e.g., picking up the spoon, placing spoon in the child's mouth) to insure that the food gets to the child's mouth so that she can be given positive reinforcement (e.g., playing with a toy, verbal praise) for taking a bite. It also means that the child cannot avoid eating by simply refusing it. The authors indicate that by combining reinforcement with the forced feeding, the forced feeding is limited to being "educational" and a means to an end (i.e., independent eating) rather than simply providing food for survival. This forced feeding involves only placing food in a child's mouth

Chapter 8: Behavioral Feeding Problems, continued

when she is in an upright position (making aspiration unlikely and giving the child the choice to expel or swallow the food).

Vibration to Decrease Tactile Defensiveness

Shaefer (1960) first demonstrated vibration generated by an electric toothbrush to be a reinforcing stimulus for pill taking in children. Rehagen and Thelen (1972) found that vibration was reinforcing to a significant degree in ambulatory severely and moderately retarded children. It has also been shown to be a stronger reinforcer than food (Johnson et al., 1978). Vibration, however, is not a universal reinforcer and when the stimulation stops, the responses may die away (Jones, 1980).

Peter Dennison, a feeding specialist in New Zealand, documents using vibration of the Broxodent® electric toothbrush (uses 50 cycles per second) to alter biting, gagging, and tactile defensiveness that may be present in children with feeding disorders. He has had considerable success using the following techniques:

- Introduce the toothbrush away from the bathroom and from any setting that could be considered "clinical."

- The introduction should be fun and non-stressful for the child.

- Try using the toothbrush before lunch as this appears to improve eating.

- Show the child how the toothbrush turns on and off.

- Start by touching the toothbrush to different parts of the child's body. Gradually work towards the head in a non-threatening manner.

- After you demonstrate to the child how she can place the toothbrush on her tongue, let her try to place it on her tongue and then bite down on it.

- Vibration can be conducted 5-10 minutes per day.

Decreasing Ruminative Vomiting

An estimated 8-10% of children and adults with developmental disorders may present with ruminative vomiting (i.e., regurgitation, rechewing, and reswallowing of previously consumed food in a repetitive manner) (Luiselli et al., 1993). Increasing food quantities (Johnston and Greene, 1992), increasing caloric density (Johnston et al., 1991), and changing the consistency of food (Rast et al., 1988) can all affect rumination frequency.

Chapter 8: Behavioral Feeding Problems, continued

In the Johnston et al. study, three mentally retarded individuals residing in an institutional facility were given meals that had gradually increasing caloric density over normal levels by adding oils, sugars, and Polycose® (a caloric supplement in the form of tasteless powder mixed with food). The results showed that although some high caloric density meals resulted in the same amount of ruminative vomiting as seen after regular calorie meals, there was an overall decrease in ruminating. The decrease was evidenced by an increase in the number of days with fewer episodes or no ruminating. It was also noted that the effects of the high calories reduced the ruminating after the meal that followed the one where the caloric density had been increased. Any such caloric alteration should be made only with the input of the primary care physician and a qualified dietician. An additional strategy to reduce ruminative vomiting is differential reinforcement, using extinction to decrease the episodes of vomiting and positive reinforcement to reward eating (Iwata et al., 1982).

Increasing Texture
The transition from bottle or breast to different textures may be the point at which feeding problems arise. For information on prevention of difficulties, refer to the section on education to prevent problems (page 186). For specifics on the transition from one texture to the next, refer to Chapter 5, pages 154-155. Basic knowledge of behavioral management strategies as outlined above can certainly help achieve the transition or eliminate minor problems (e.g., mildly restricted diet) before more significant problems (e.g., inadequate growth) develop.

Behavioral Feeding Disorders and Families

Parental factors as a cause of feeding disorders

McCann et al. (1994) indicate that some children with poor weight gain and concomitant behavioral feeding disorders come from families who have higher levels of dietary restraint and that, despite the child's low weight, their mothers restrict the child's intake of foods judged to be sweet or fattening. Family dysfunction has been found to be an indicator of chronic growth retardation, including behaviors that lead to lack of organization and planning for mealtimes (Heptinstall et al., 1987). Similarly, a caregiver's psychological difficulties, stress, and an impaired mother-child relationship are associated with a child's inadequate weight gain (Lachenmeyer, 1995).

Parents may inadvertently maintain inappropriate feeding behaviors because of their own fears about having a chronically ill child. Singer (1990) reports

Chapter 8: Behavioral Feeding Problems, continued

situations where mothers of children with cystic fibrosis felt they shouldn't curtail inappropriate feeding behaviors because of fear that their children would die.

Impact of the disorder on the family

A child with a feeding problem will inevitably have an impact on her family. The impact can be considerable for families who have a child with a feeding tube (and these children will also often have multiple medical diagnoses). The impact may be less significant if the problem is a restricted diet or "battles" at mealtimes.

Remediation of a feeding problem must include the family at all stages if the program is to succeed, and it must be sensitive to individual family dynamics, learning strategies, and expectations. Parrish (1997) writes of families with children with chronic illnesses/disabilities (e.g., a feeding disorder) as experiencing the stages of grief delineated by Kubler-Ross (1969):

- denial
- anger
- depression
- disorganization
- eventual adaptation or coping

Mothers frequently blame themselves for their children's inadequate weight gain (McCann et al., 1994), although Lachenmeyer (1995) states that the effective caregiver is not one whose "whole sense of self is based on whether and how much the child eats."

Numerous issues may also arise in families whose children present with a feeding disorder (e.g., excessive sibling rivalry, marital difficulty, financial strains). Much of our culture's socialization revolves around food (e.g., birthdays, holidays, family gatherings) and feeding problems may make normal socialization complicated or impossible. Families need to be able to explain their children's condition to others, (e.g., teachers, peers, or neighbors). In addition, parents must maintain a balance between allowing their children to be appropriately social with their peers and protecting their children to some extent from social stigma and teasing, particularly on the part of other children (Parrish, 1997).

The feeding specialist needs to be sensitive to family dynamics so that appropriate referrals can be made to other professionals (e.g., social workers) as needed.

Working with Children Who Take Nothing by Mouth (NPO)

Physicians may not refer a child who is NPO with only tube feeding to the SLP until the child is ready to transition to oral feeding. This is unfortunate because children who do not have the opportunity to develop oral-motor skills and who do not learn the feeling of normal hunger or satiation will have a more difficult time

Chapter 8: Behavioral Feeding Problems, continued

making the transition to oral feeding when it is safe to do so (Orr and Allen, 1986).

Physicians may think that the only thing an SLP does is introduce food and work on "feeding." Therapy should begin with infants who are tube fed to prepare them for later oral feeding. The eventual outcome of such intervention may be successful feeding, but the intervention is targeted towards developing the appropriate use of the mouth, respiratory, and phonatory systems in exploration and sound play (Morris and Klein, 1987).

Treatment Techniques for the Non-oral Infant or Child

1. Oral-motor treatment: See Chapters 5 and 6 for information on specifics of treatment.

2. Desensitization: Children who have undergone numerous invasive procedures (e.g., placement of NG tube, suctioning, bronchoscopy) may develop a conditioned aversion to swallowing (Di Scipio et al., 1978). This aversion may continue long after the invasive procedures have been eliminated. Treatment must be directed toward decreasing sensitivity through positive interaction between the child and the therapist (e.g., talking, touching, holding) so that the child does not see the therapist as a provider of more aversive stimuli (Morris and Klein, 1987). This interaction is particularly important during non-oral feeding times to simulate normal feeding procedures. The child's mother, a nurse, or another significant other can also perform desensitization (Senez et al., 1996).

3. Tactile stimulation to move the threshold of the gag reflex posteriorly if the child has a hyperactive gag (See page 153.)

4. Gustatory and olfactory stimulation to desensitize the child to the taste and smell of food. Placing a finger with breast milk or formula on the infant's tongue or a variety of other flavors for older children can do this (Senez et al., 1996)

5. Regulated feeding times to establish the rhythms of sleep and activity, hunger and satiation, and empty and full stomach (Senez et al., 1996)

Transition from Tube Feeding to PO Intake

Children may be referred for a feeding assessment as a result of the desire to terminate tube feeding. There are numerous reasons for the presence of the tube (e.g., prematurity, anatomical problem, neurological disorder). It may be that the child no longer presents with the medical reason for the tube (e.g., anatomical problem surgically corrected), but because of lack of experience/skill, the child is unable to make a smooth transition to oral feeding without some assistance from a feeding specialist.

Chapter 8: Behavioral Feeding Problems, *continued*

Children who return to feeding by mouth prior to the developmental age of 6 months often make a smoother transition than those who for one reason or another do not make the transition until later (Blackman and Nelson, 1985). The reason frequently cited for this is that they miss a "critical period" of food acceptance/tolerance making introduction extremely difficult (Illingsworth and Lister, 1964). Orr and Allen (1986) indicate that the severity of a feeding problem and the length of time of non-oral feeding are positively correlated. That is, the longer a child lacks oral feeding, the more severe the feeding problem will become. Senez et al. (1996) discuss the importance of early feeding to integrate the oropharyngeal zone into the body pattern which is then recorded in the cortical sensorimotor areas. The hypothesis is that, in children who are tube fed, certain areas of the brain don't develop fully and, therefore, are not sensitive to impulses from the oropharyngeal zone.

Transition from non-oral to oral feeding needs to be planned carefully to assure success. The feeding specialist must be involved before tube feedings are terminated, not after the fact when the child may be exhibiting problems. Prerequisites for transition to oral feeding are:

- The child is medically stable.

- The child can swallow without significant risk of aspiration.

- If solid food is to be introduced, make sure the child is at the developmental age the pediatrician recommends for introducing solids (some say 4 months, some say 6 months).

- Begin with a period of desensitization if the child has been the subject of a variety of aversive oral stimuli.

The first stage of transition that Blackman and Nelson (1985) name and describe as the **preparation stage** involves the following three steps:

1. For children who get continuous tube feeding, the tube feeding schedule should be altered so that it approximates the times for oral feeding (three meals and two snacks) to coincide with the rest of the family. Doing this helps the child get used to the timing of the upcoming oral feedings and reinforces the social nature of eating. For some families, this may not only require adjustment for the child, but for the family as a whole if social eating has not been a regular event.

2. Changes need to be made to the formula to make it as standard as possible. Blackman and Nelson suggest that standard cow's milk or soy-based formula are preferable to "pre-digested" preparations.

3. The child needs to be receiving sufficient calories to maintain growth. A registered dietitian can help with this.

Chapter 8: Behavioral Feeding Problems, continued

Once the preparation stage is complete (it may take a few days or a few weeks), treatment can be initiated as part of the **transition stage**. The following should be considered, dependent on the child's tolerance of oral feeding (See Chapter 10 for specific goals.):

- Add oral feedings to tube-fed mealtimes, gradually starting with very small amounts of liquids and solids.

- To rule out food allergies, it is necessary to try only one new food item at a time for a period of 3 to 4 days as one would with a normal child transitioning to different textures. Food allergies can also be assessed by placing new foods in pureed form and diluted with water through the tube at similar intervals (Morris and Klein, 1987). This allows for allergic reactions without the child making a connection to oral feeding that might jeopardize progress with an oral diet.

- Give the child spoons, bowls, and food to play with to encourage the child to become comfortable with food and utensils (Morris and Klein, 1987).

- Elicit a lot of verbal praise during eating. This should be a "no pressure" situation. Depending on the child's ability to chew, this may be a good time to introduce foods such as pudding, yogurt, cookies, crackers, dry cereal, or cheese. These foods should be easy and "fun" to eat, which will encourage the lack of pressure.

- Negative behaviors should essentially be ignored although verbalizing "No!" is legitimate in extreme cases, as is gentle restraint to reduce self-injury and to establish the adult's control of the situation (Dunbar et al., 1990).

- Set a time limit of 15-30 minutes for oral feeding. The remainder of the meal should then be fed via the tube.

- If a child demonstrates avoidance or fighting behaviors in response to oral feedings, provide a break between the attempted oral feeding and the tube feeding (Morris and Klein, 1987). Otherwise the tube feeding may be regarded as the "easy way out" by the child and reinforce the fighting/avoidance behaviors. That is, giving the tube feeding right away may reinforce the unwanted behavior.

- Early in the period of transition, it may become apparent that the child has particular times of day when she is more ready to eat by mouth, although she may still be getting the majority of her calories non-orally. If so, give a reduced amount of food in the tube-fed meal prior to a planned oral meal to increase hunger for the oral meal (Morris and Klein, 1987). Providing an oral snack prior to an anticipated non-oral meal may also take advantage of hunger, particularly as the amounts of non-oral feedings are reduced.

Chapter 8: Behavioral Feeding Problems, continued

- Once the child is able to take the majority of calories by mouth, tube feeding can be diluted by 75% and then gradually tapered off. At this stage, the child may need a small amount of tube feeding to provide 100% of needed calories (a dietician can help with the calculations). So as not to invalidate the child's new found success of oral feeding, it may be possible to make up the additional calories at nap time or at night when the child is less aware of the process of tube feeding (Morris and Klein, 1987). This should be done with care so as not to interfere with the newly established hunger cycles and to make sure the child doesn't feel that she is a "failure" because she is using the tube, or that it is an easy way out from eating food orally.

- If feeding has already become something of a battle between the child and the caregiver, it may be necessary to remove the caregiver temporarily from feeding so the emotional stress already present does not negatively impact upon the new approach (Dunbar et al., 1990).

- Children should be transitioned to as normal and varied a diet as possible. Inevitably there will be some individual preferences. Something to consider is that children who have been fed non-orally may prefer spicier foods (Arvedson, 1993). Spicier foods serve to alert a system that has not been used to food.

Once the transition from tube feeding to oral feeding has been successfully made, the next step is removal of the feeding tube. This should not be done in haste. Leaving the tube an additional few weeks or possibly months is not a problem unless infection is a concern. The child should be given enough time (around 6 months) to stabilize oral feeding skills and preferably go through an illness when the need for non-oral feeding may arise.

Children with head injuries may have some difficulty transitioning from tube to oral feeding. Waiting until the period of extreme agitation has passed to remove feeding tubes may be warranted to achieve an easier transition to oral intake. It is important to avoid forced feeding as well as any additional parental anxiety. Progress may be slow (Ylvisaker and Weinstein, 1989).

When an Inpatient Program Is Needed

Treatment for behavioral feeding problems can be conducted on an inpatient basis, an outpatient basis, or a combination of the two. The type and the severity of the disorder and the child and family dynamics will determine the type of intervention, with the least intrusive intervention being the goal (Arvedson, 1997). Although much feeding therapy can be achieved very adequately on an outpatient basis, there are some children who may benefit greatly from an inpatient program, particularly when outpatient therapy has not achieved established goals.

Chapter 8: Behavioral Feeding Problems, continued

Dunbar et al. (1990) provide an excellent list of reasons which may lead to the consideration of an inpatient intensive feeding program:

- Extreme stress experienced by parents over failed efforts to achieve adequate oral feeding

- Failed attempts by professionals and parents to make changes in feeding behaviors when treatment has been conducted on an outpatient basis

- Inability of parents to bring a child to therapy due to distance, economics, work schedules, or transportation

- The need for medical monitoring during the process of being weaned from tube feeding

- Availability of team involvement

- Treatment timelines as specified by third party payers

Singer (1987) reported that children from the most deprived families may be referred for inpatient hospitalizations more frequently than other groups, and they also tend to be those who are subsequently placed in welfare custody. Inpatient programs can have some very positive outcomes such as reducing family stress by improving confidence in parenting skills as the parents return to being primary feeders and improving parent-child interaction (Dunbar et al., 1990).

Treating a child with a behavioral feeding disorder can be challenging. A thorough evaluation and careful analysis of all contributing factors is essential to establish and implement an effective treatment plan.

Chapter 8: Behavioral Feeding Problems, *continued*

Example Food Diary

Child: ___Takisha___

Date	Time Beg./End	Location (e.g., kitchen)	Location of child (e.g., high chair)	People Present (e.g., mom, sister, friend)	Who fed? (e.g., child, mom)	Types of food given	Responses to types of food	Amount eaten (e.g., 1 piece pizza, 3 crackers, 4 grapes)	Problem behaviors noted during meal (e.g., wouldn't open mouth for spoon)	Your reaction to problem behavior
10/15	8:00-8:10	kitchen	standing by table	mom, brother	child	Cream of Wheat®, crackers, juice	spit out ⟩⟩	0 2 1 box	spitting	held head and gave another spoonful
10/15	6:00-6:20	"	"	mom, dad, brother	child & mom	macaroni & cheese, juice	ate some ⟩	2 tsp. 2 boxes	very small bites	ignored
10/16	9:30-9:45	"	"	mom	mom	cereal, Ensure®, juice	shut mouth ⟩⟩	0 1 can 2 boxes	refused cereal, threw spoon	didn't feel like fighting

Completed by: _____

Chapter 8: Behavioral Feeding Problems, *continued*

Food Diary

Child: _____

Date	Time Beg. /End	Location (e.g., kitchen)	Location of child (e.g., high chair)	People Present (e.g., mom, sister, friend)	Who fed? (e.g., child, mom)	Types of food given	Responses to types of food	Amount eaten (e.g., 1 piece pizza, 3 crackers, 4 grapes)	Problem behaviors noted during meal (e.g., wouldn't open mouth for spoon)	Your reaction to problem behavior

Completed by: _____

Chapter 8: Behavioral Feeding Problems, continued

Example Observation of Eating

Child: _Takisha_

SLP: _NS_

Date: _10-27-98_

Position during feeding:

___ Reclined

_✓_ Seating device: _____

___ Sitting unsupported

Foods Presented (Describe Taste & Texture)	Temperature	How Presented? (C)up (SP)oon (ST)raw (F)inger	Fed by? (C)hild (P)arent	What did child do with food?	Child's response to caregiver	Caregiver's response to child
oatmeal	warm	SP	P	spit out	pushes hand away	holds hand & forces spoon in
cracker	room temp	F	C	bites through & lets it dissolve	n/a	no encouragement given
cheese	cold	F	C	very small bite put in cheek	n/a	"Take a bigger piece."

Chapter 8: Behavioral Feeding Problems, *continued*

Observation of Eating

Child: _____   Date: _____

SLP: _____

Position during feeding:

_____ Reclined

_____ Seating device: _____

_____ Sitting unsupported

Foods Presented (Describe Taste & Texture)	Temperature	How Presented? (C)up (SP)oon (ST)raw (F)inger	Fed by? (C)hild (P)arent	What did child do with food?	Child's response to caregiver	Caregiver's response to child

Chapter 8: Behavioral Feeding Problems, continued

Appendix 8-A

Ways to Prevent or Minimize Feeding Problems
(Taking the Stress Out of Mealtimes)

Caregiver Do's

Do turn off the television.

Do accept that it's okay for all children to miss a meal once in a while.

Do praise children with words when they meet your expectations for eating a meal (e.g., "You did a great job eating your breakfast!" "I'm proud of you for eating those carrots!").

Do offer a variety of foods at each meal and across meals. Offering the same food (e.g., peanut butter and jelly sandwiches) will make a child less likely to accept new foods later.

Do limit snacks. One snack between meals (e.g., middle of the morning, middle of the afternoon) is okay, but if a child snacks throughout the day, he/she will never develop hunger to eat a complete, more balanced meal.

Do provide healthy nutritious snacks (e.g., fruit, cheese, crackers) to create a solid basis for nutrition later.

Do limit juice intake as this can reduce the desire to eat.

Do make mealtimes a time when the family gets together, even if it's only once a day. This takes the stress away from eating for the sake of eating and encourages the social nature of meals.

Do accept that most children like sweet foods and that such foods are okay in moderation.

Do give small portions. This increases the likelihood that a child will be successful. It is always easier to ask for more.

Do establish mealtime rules like sitting in a chair and using a fork and spoon. Reward with words when a child follows the rules (e.g., "I'm so pleased you sat in your chair while you were eating."). Invite children to help establish the rules.

Do accept that meals make a mess. Fill cups 1/4 - 1/2 full. Put a plastic mat under the child's plate and make sure that all surfaces can be washed easily (i.e., avoid upholstered chairs). Keeping a hand-held vacuum handy is helpful. Involve children in the clean-up process whenever possible.

Do keep trying new foods with a child. Just because he/she declines them one week doesn't mean he/she won't eat them two weeks later.

Do provide a good role model for eating balanced meals at regular intervals.

Do ignore inappropriate mealtime behaviors (unless the child is in danger) as this may reduce the child's willingness to use them to get something he/she wants (e.g., cheese instead of fruit).

The Source for Pediatric Dysphagia

Chapter 8: Behavioral Feeding Problems, continued

Appendix 8-A, continued

Ways to Prevent or Minimize Feeding Problems
(Taking the Stress Out of Mealtimes)

Caregiver Don'ts

Don't force a child to eat what he/she doesn't want to. This can develop into a battle of wills.

Don't offer alternate food when the child has declined what is on his/her plate.

Don't give a child extra attention because he/she won't eat.

Don't coax a child to eat (e.g., "If you eat three more bites, you can watch Barney later.").

Don't allow the child to get down from the table because he/she doesn't want to eat.

Don't punish the child for not eating.

Don't allow a child to graze by coming to the table throughout a meal, taking food, and walking around with it. This leads to a long and drawn out meal with little structure from beginning to end.

Don't give dessert unless the child has eaten the amount of food on his/her plate agreed to at the beginning of the meal.

Chapter 8: Behavioral Feeding Problems, continued

Appendix 8-B

Information About Feeding Therapy

The following information may be useful to help you understand what you can do to help your child be a more successful eater. You are an important team player because you know your child best of all!

During your child's feeding evaluation, the feeding specialist (most likely a speech-language pathologist) collected a great deal of information about your child. You may have started to be more aware of how, what, and when your child eats, or doesn't eat. Using the information you provided, and by addressing your concerns and the strengths and weaknesses of your child, the feeding specialist will suggest areas that need to be addressed in therapy. These will become your child's "goals." Your feeding specialist will then make a treatment plan to create steps to reach these goals.

Your feeding specialist may have talked to you about ways to change some of the behaviors that your child exhibits during feeding. There are several different ways to change a child's behaviors to achieve the goals that have been established. The most common way is the use of "behavioral techniques." Ask your feeding specialist how you can best help your child with these techniques. It is important that your child is being taught the same things in the same way (even by different people). Otherwise the child may get confused about what is expected of him/her.

The following is a list of techniques that your child's feeding specialist may use:

- **Reinforcement** means that as a result of something a child is doing (his/her behavior), we do something (reinforce) to make it more likely that the behavior will happen again.

- **Positive reinforcement** is the easiest form of reinforcement. It means that when a child behaves in a certain way, we provide something that is favorable or positive for the child. For example, we can provide positive reinforcement with words like, "You're doing a great job eating your cereal!" We have positively reinforced the behavior of eating cereal, which makes it more likely that next time the child eats cereal, he/she will also do a good job with it.

    We can provide positive reinforcement with words and actions. "I'm so proud of you that you stayed in your chair while we ate supper. Give me five!" We have positively reinforced the child's behavior of sitting at the table.

    We can positively reinforce with rewards. "You did such a good job eating all the food on your plate. Now you can have dessert." We have positively reinforced eating the amount of food we want the child to eat.

- **Negative reinforcement** involves taking away something that is a "negative" for the child. Taking the negative away makes it more likely that the behavior that occurs before the negative is taken away will happen more often. For

Chapter 8: Behavioral Feeding Problems, continued

Information About Feeding Therapy, continued

example, eating green beans may be something that is a "negative" for the child. If the child is given five green beans and told that once he/she has eaten all five, he/she will not be expected to eat any more green beans at that meal (i.e., We have taken away the demand to eat more green beans.), we are negatively reinforcing eating green beans.

Another example involves using a timer during a meal. Set a timer at the beginning of a meal and tell the child that he/she may not get down from the table until the timer goes off. This uses negative reinforcement. Sitting at the table is a negative for the child. The timer going off releases the child from the situation.

- **Modeling** provides opportunities for children to learn by imitating their parents, siblings, or anyone else they see. By watching what, how, and when other people eat, children learn what is expected of them. By setting a good example of eating balanced meals, not eating excessive amounts of snack foods, using utensils, sitting at the table, talking at mealtimes instead of watching television, and cleaning up after meals, family members can model appropriate behaviors. If we want the child to stay in his/her booster seat at the table while eating and we eat walking around the kitchen and talking on the phone, we are sending mixed messages about our expectations.

- **Shaping** involves taking what may be a very difficult behavior for a child and making it easier by breaking it down into smaller steps. For example, a child may be overwhelmed when asked to eat a "normal-sized" helping of cereal. By offering a very small amount and then gradually increasing the size of the helping over the next few days or weeks, we have "shaped" a behavior.

- **Antecedent manipulation** involves changing what happens immediately before a behavior we don't want in an attempt to get rid of that behavior. For example, if a child does not like the food items on his/her plate to touch each other and throws a tantrum or refuses to eat when it happens, we can manipulate what happens before the problem (not letting the foods touch by using a plate divided into sections), so the child will not behave inappropriately.

Your child's feeding specialist will work with you so you can learn to use these behavior modification techniques. By working together, you can help improve your child's eating behavior.

Chapter 8: Behavioral Feeding Problems, continued

References

Ament, P. "Removal of Gagging: A Response to Variable Behavior Patterns." *The International Journal of Clinical and Experimental Hypnosis*, Vol. 19, No. 1, 1971, pp. 1-9.

Arvedson, J. "Behavioral Issues and Implications with Pediatric Feeding Disorders." *Seminars in Speech and Language*, Vol. 18, No. 1, 1997, pp. 51-70.

Atkins, L. et al. "A Multimodal Approach to Functional Dysphagia." *Journal of the American Academy of Child and Adolescent Psychiatry*, Vol. 33, No. 7, 1994, pp. 1012-1016.

Babbitt, R. et al. "Behavioral Feeding Disorders." In Tuchman, D. and Walter, R. (eds.) *Disorders of Feeding and Swallowing in Infants and Children*, San Diego: Singular Publishing Group, Inc., 1994, pp. 77-95.

Bithoney, W.G. and Rathburn, J.M. "Failure to Thrive." In Levine, M.D. (ed.) *Developmental Behavioral Pediatrics*, Philadelphia: W.B. Saunders, 1983.

Blackman, J. and Nelson, C. "Reinstituting Oral Feedings in Children Fed by Gastrostomy Tube." *Clinical Pediatrics*, Vol. 24, No. 8, 1985, pp. 434-438.

Carstens, C. "Behavioral Treatment of Functional Dysphagia in a 12-Year-Old Boy." *Psychosomatics*, Vol. 23, No. 2, 1982, pp. 195-196.

Cooper, L. et al. "Use of Component Analyses to Identify Variables in Treatment Packages for Children with Feeding Disorders." *Journal of Applied Behavior Analysis*, Vol. 28, 1995, pp. 139-153.

Culbert, T. et al. "Hypnobehavioral Approaches for School-Age Children with Dysphagia and Food Aversion: A Case Series." *Developmental and Behavioral Pediatrics*, Vol. 17, No. 5, 1996, pp. 335-341.

Dahl, M. and Bristiansson, B. "Early Feeding Problems in an Affluent Society." *Acta Paediatrica Scandinavica*, Vol. 76, 1987, pp. 881-888.

Davis, L.F. "Some Keys for Primary Caregivers." In Perske, R. (ed.) *Mealtimes for Severely and Profoundly Handicapped Persons: New Concepts and Attitudes*, Baltimore: University Park Press, 1977, pp. 27-31.

Dennison, P. (Public Health Dentist). "The Use of Vibration to Favourably Modify the Gag and Bite Reflexes and Tactile Defensiveness," Desktop Publication via Worldwide Web, 1998.

DiScipio, W.J. et al. "Traumatically Acquired Conditioned Dysphagia in Children." *Annals of Otology, Rhinology, and Laryngology*, Vol. 87, 1978, pp. 509-514.

Dunbar, S. et al. "The Transition from Non-oral to Oral Feeding in Children." *The American Journal of Occupational Therapy*, Vol. 45, No. 5, 1991, pp. 402-408.

Chapter 8: Behavioral Feeding Problems, continued

Finney, J. "Preventing Common Feeding Problems: Prevention in Primary Care." *Pediatric Clinics of North America*, Vol. 33, No. 4, 1986, pp. 775-788.

Frischmeyer, P. and Millard, T. "Use of Component Analyses to Identify Active Variables in Treatment Packages for Children with Feeding Disorders." *Journal of Applied Behavior Analysis*, Vol. 28, 1995, pp. 139-153.

Geertsma, A. et al. "Feeding Resistance After Parenteral Hyperalimentation." *American Journal of Diseases in Children*, Vol. 139, 1985, pp. 255-256.

Handen, B. et al. "Feeding Induction in Children Who Refuse to Eat." *American Journal of Diseases in Children*, Vol. 140, 1986, pp. 52-54.

Heptinstall, E. et al. "Nutrition and Mealtime Behavior in Families of Growth-Retarded Children." *Human Nutrition: Applied Nutrition*, Vol. 41A, 1987, pp. 390-402.

Hoch, T. et al. "A Swallow Induction Avoidance Procedure to Establish Eating." *Journal of Behavior Therapy and Experimental Psychiatry*, Vol. 26, No. 1, 1995, pp. 41-50.

Hoch, T. et al. "Contingency Contacting — Combining Positive Reinforcement and Escape Extinction Procedures to Treat Persistent Food Refusal." *Behavior Modification*, Vol. 18, 1994, pp. 106-128.

Illingsworth, R. and Lister, J. "The Critical or Sensitive Period with Special Reference to Certain Feeding Problems in Infants and Children." *The Journal of Pediatrics*, Vol. 65, 1964, pp. 839-848.

Iwata, B. et al. "Pediatric Feeding Disorders: Behavioral Analysis and Treatment." In Accardo, P. (ed.) *Failure to Thrive in Infancy and Early Childhood*, Baltimore: University Park Press, 1982, pp. 297-329.

Johnson, D. et al. "Vibration and Praise as Reinforcers for Mentally Handicapped People." *Mental Retardation*, Vol. 16, 1978, pp. 339-342.

Johnston, J.M. and Greene, K. "Relation Between Ruminating and Quantity of Food Consumed." *Mental Retardation*, Vol. 30, No. 1, 1992, pp. 7-11.

Johnston, J.M. et al. "Effects of Caloric Level on Ruminating." *Journal of Applied Behavior Analysis*, Vol. 24, No. 3, 1991, pp. 597-603.

Jolley, S.G. et al. "Pharyngeal and Swallowing Disorders in Infants." *Seminars in Pediatric Surgery*, Vol. 4, No. 3, 1995, pp. 157-165.

Jones, C. "The Uses of Mechanical Vibration with the Severely Mentally Handicapped." *Mental Handicap*, Vol. 8, 1980, pp. 112-114.

Kubler-Ross, E. *On Death and Dying*, New York: Macmillan, 1969.

Chapter 8: Behavioral Feeding Problems, continued

Lachenmeyer, J. "Behavior Aspects of Feeding Disorders." In Rosenthal, S. et al. (eds.) *Dysphagia and the Child with Developmental Disabilities*, San Diego: Singular Publishing Group, Inc., 1995, pp. 143-153.

Luiselli, J.K. et al. "Evaluation of a Behavioral Medicine Consultative Treatment for Chronic, Ruminative Vomiting." *Journal of Behavior Therapy and Experimental Psychiatry*, Vol. 24, No. 1, 1993, pp. 27-35.

Madsen, H. et al. "Increasing Rural Head Start Children's Consumption of Middle-Class Meals." *Journal of Applied Behavior Analysis*, Vol. 7, No. 2, 1974, pp. 257-262.

McCann, J. et al. "Eating Habits and Attitudes of Mothers of Children with Non-organic Failure to Thrive." *Archives of Disease at Childhood*, Vol. 70, 1964, pp. 234-236.

Morris, S.E. and Klein, M.D. *Pre-Feeding Skills*, San Antonio: Communication Skill Builders, a division of The Psychological Corporation, 1987, pp. 270-286, 319-335.

O'Neil, P.M. et al. "Controlling Childhood Rumination Through Differential Reinforcement of Other Behavior." *Behavior Modification*, Vol. 3, No. 3, 1979, pp. 355-372.

Orr, M.J. and Allen, S. "Optimal Oral Experiences for Infants on Long-Term Total Parenteral Nutrition." *Nutrition in Clinical Practice*, Vol. 6, 1986, pp. 288-295.

Palmer, S. et al. "Applied Behavior Analysis in the Treatment of Childhood Feeding Problems." *Developmental Medicine and Child Neurology*, Vol. 17, 1975, pp. 333-339.

Parrish, M. "Family Adaptation to a Child's Feeding and Swallowing Disorder: A Social Work Perspective." *Seminars in Speech and Language*, Vol. 18, No. 1, 1997, pp. 71-78.

Parsons, M.B. & Reid, D.H. "Assessing Food Preferences Among Persons with Profound Mental Retardation: Providing Opportunities to Make Choices." *Journal of Applied Behavioral Analysis*, Vol. 23, 1990, pp. 183-195.

Payne, P. and Sheppard, J. "School-Based Programming for Managing Food Refusal with Tube-Fed Children." Presentation at New Jersey Speech-Language-Hearing Association Convention, 1998.

Ramsay, M. et al. "Non-organic Failure to Thrive: Growth Failure Secondary to Feeding-Skills Disorder." *Developmental Medicine and Child Neurology*, Vol. 35, 1993, pp. 285-297.

Rast, J. et al. "Effects of Pre-meal Chewing on Ruminative Behavior." *American Journal of Mental Retardation*, Vol. 93, No. 1, 1988, pp. 67-74.

Rehagen, N. and Thelen, M. "Vibration as Positive Reinforcement for Retarded Children." *Journal of Abnormal Psychology*, Vol. 80, No. 2, 1972, pp. 162-167.

Chapter 8: Behavioral Feeding Problems, continued

Riordan, M. et al. "Behavioral Treatment of Food Refusal and Selectivity in Developmentally Disabled Children." *Applied Research in Mental Retardation*, Vol. 93, No. 1, 1980, pp. 95-112.

Senez, C. et al. "Weaning Children from Tube to Oral Feeding." *Child's Nervous System*, Vol. 12, 1996, pp. 590-594.

Shaefer, H. "Vibration as a Reinforcer with Infant Children." *Journal of Experimental Analysis of Behavior*, Vol. 3, 1960, p. 160.

Singer, L. "Long-Term Hospitalization of Nonorganic Failure-to-Thrive Infants: Patient Characteristics and Hospital Course." *Developmental and Behavioral Pediatrics*, Vol. 8, 1987, pp. 25-31.

Singer, L. "When a Sick Child Won't — or Can't — Eat." *Contemporary Pediatrics*, Vol. 7, 1990, pp. 60-75.

Singer, L. et al. "Cognitive-Behavioral Treatment of Health-Impairing Food Phobias in Children." *Journal of the American Academy of Child and Adolescent Psychiatry*, Vol. 31, No. 5, 1992, pp. 847-852.

Smith, M. and Lifshitz, F. "Excess Fruit Juice Consumption as a Contributing Factor in Nonorganic Failure to Thrive." *Pediatrics*, Vol. 93, No. 3, 1994, pp. 438-443.

Stein, A. and Fairburn, C. "Children of Mothers with Bulimia Nervosa." *British Medical Journal*, Vol. 229, 1989, pp. 777-778.

Walco, G. "A Behavioral Treatment for Difficulty in Swallowing Pills." *Journal of Behavior Therapy and Experimental Psychiatry*, Vol. 17, No. 2, 1986, pp. 127-128.

Wilcox, W.D. et al. "Failure to Thrive — A Continuing Problem of Definition." *Clinical Pediatrics*, Vol. 28, No. 9, 1989, pp. 391-394.

Ylvisaker, M. and Weinstein, M. "Recovery of Oral Feeding After Pediatric Head Injury." *Journal of Head Trauma Rehabilitation*, Vol. 4, 1989, pp. 51-63.

Chapter 9: Drooling

Drooling is most often seen in children with cerebral palsy, mental retardation, or other neurological or neuromuscular disorders. It can also be seen in healthy children, even beyond the age of five years. Drooling can have significant negative effects on the child including:

- physical: the child may have a chapped face and may also transmit infectious diseases

- social: the child's peers may not want to interact with him because of the child's wet face and clothing

- psychological: the child may develop poor self-esteem and lack of self-confidence because of the social impact of the drooling

Anatomy and Physiology of Drooling

Brodsky (1984) provides an excellent description of the anatomy, physiology, and pathophysiology of drooling. Readers are referred to this reference for more detailed information, particularly concerning surgical intervention. Brodsky reports that approximately one liter of saliva is produced per day. It is mostly produced by three pairs of major salivary glands and other minor salivary glands:

- parotid glands (located in the soft tissues of the cheek) produce about 30% of the volume; mostly thin secretions

- sub-mandibular glands (located in the sub-mandibular triangle in the neck) produce between 50-70% of saliva production; somewhat more viscous secretions

- sub-lingual glands (located on the floor of the mouth) account for 5% of saliva production; predominantly mucoid secretions

- minor salivary glands (located throughout the mucosa of the palate and oral cavity) produce the rest of the saliva

Functions of Saliva

Saliva is necessary to moisten food to help with chewing and swallowing. It also contains enzymes that begin the breakdown of foods for digestion. Saliva also provides some protection from dental disease and oral infection, as well as aiding in articulation. It is very difficult to articulate accurately if the mucosa of the oral cavity is dry.

Too Much Saliva?

Rarely is having too much saliva the cause of severe drooling. However some things can contribute to increased production of saliva. Those include:

Chapter 9: Drooling, *continued*

- dental caries
- gingivitis
- disorders of malocclusion
- medications such as tranquilizers or anti-convulsants. These may result in the increase in the amount of saliva produced or a reduction in the ability to swallow frequently enough to control the secretions.

Factors that Increase Severity of Drooling

Some factors may make the severity of drooling worse, including:

- a child's inability to maintain good body posture

- airway obstruction, which requires open mouth breathing posture

- decreased oral sensation

- reduced ability to concentrate and remember to swallow

Interdisciplinary Assessment

Brodsky points out the importance of an interdisciplinary assessment for cases of severe drooling because of the many factors concerning the cause and possible treatments for drooling. Recommended specialists to participate on a team and their functions include:

- Speech-Language Pathologist: completes an evaluation of oral-motor function and swallowing and assessment of cognitive-communicative and language skills to help determine if the child will be able to follow directions

- Dentist: assesses the gums, teeth, and occlusal relationship. Dental caries are a common cause of increased salivation, and Arvedson (1993) reports that once severe dental caries have been treated, very often the saliva decreases and the drooling problem is resolved. In addition, if the child has a severe malocclusion (open bite) and has accompanying decreased tone and strength in the lips, he may lose saliva anteriorly.

- Otolaryngologist: assesses upper airway. Enlarged adenoids or allergies which result in chronic rhinitis may cause the child to mouth breathe with an open mouth posture. Enlarged tonsils can also have an effect on the ability to control secretions.

- Neurologist: assesses any related or causative neurological disorders

- Physical Therapist: assesses total body control, trunk control, etc.

Chapter 9: Drooling, *continued*

Assessing Oral-Motor Function, Swallowing, and Drooling

Any child referred for excessive drooling should receive a complete oral-motor and swallowing evaluation. (See pages 88-112.)

In addition, information should be obtained about the following factors which may be related to the drooling, either as a cause, a contributing or exacerbating factor, or which may interfere with any planned intervention. (See Appendix 9-A, page 222.)

1. Does the child drool constantly or is it intermittent? If it is intermittent, does it seem more related to the posture the child is in, the time of day, and/or the activity the child is involved in?

2. Does the child seem aware that his face is wet? If the child does not seem at all uncomfortable with a wet face or shirt, he may lack motivation to stay dry.

3. If the child has received treatment for the drooling in the past, find out the approach that was used and what the results were.

4. Does the child breathe through his mouth or nose? If the child has to keep his mouth open to maintain an open airway, he may be less likely to want to close his mouth frequently to swallow saliva.

5. The medications a child is taking may be causing an increase in saliva or a reduction in the ability to swallow frequently enough. Typical medications with these effects are tranquilizers or anti-convulsants.

6. and 7. The child's cognitive level will have a direct impact on his ability to participate in the treatment program. If the child is not able to follow two-step commands, he may not be able to fully participate.

8. Does the child even understand the concepts of *wet* and *dry*? If not, the treatment plan cannot use a conceptual base.

9. If the child keeps his hands or toys in his mouth, drooling may be promoted because his mouth is always open.

10. How concerned is the caregiver about the problem? For some caregivers, the drooling may be their biggest worry. Their child may be teased about a wet shirt or other children may avoid playing with the child. For other caregivers, the drooling is a minor nuisance and they simply change the child's clothing frequently. If the drooling is not a big problem for the caregiver, she may not be interested in a complex behavioral management program to reduce the drooling.

Chapter 9: Drooling, continued

11. Does the child have significant dental problems? These problems may contribute to an increase in the production of saliva, and dental treatment may need to occur before a behavioral program is attempted.

Johnson and Scott's (1993) *Saliva Control Assessment Form* and *Observation of Saliva Control Checklist* gives more detailed information. They have modified several scales of severity of drooling into a *Saliva Loss Rating Scale*. Most of the scales are very similar, rating the frequency and the severity (e.g., amount) of drooling. Johnson and Scott suggest that two independent raters should fill out such scales over a period of 5-10 days.

Options for Treatment

Eliminating Related Causal Factors

1. Complete an evaluation and treat any related problems (e.g., dental problems, nasal obstructions, revisions of medications) that might be causing increased salivation.

2. If this treatment is not effective, then an oral-motor program and/or behavioral program should be instituted. These are described in more detail below and in Chapters 5 and 8. (Many of the behavior modification techniques can be applied.)

3. If an oral-motor program and/or behavioral program are not successful, then pharmacological intervention can be considered. Camp-Bruno et al. (1989) found that anti-cholinergic medications (e.g., benztropine) inhibited salivary secretions in a controlled study with 20 severe droolers. However, there are side effects of this medication including blurred vision, urinary retention, constipation, and confusion.

4. Finally, for patients who have severe problems that have not responded to other intervention techniques, surgery can be considered. Some of the salivary glands can be removed to reduce the amount of saliva secreted. Other surgeries actually reroute the saliva so it is deposited more posteriorly in the oral cavity and is swallowed more easily.

Oral-Motor and/or Behavioral Treatment Approach

Oral-Motor

After the assessment is completed and option #2 described above is chosen, then a systematic oral-motor and/or behavioral treatment approach should be instituted. Problems noted on the evaluation in positioning, head control, oral-motor control, or swallowing should be addressed as a way to improve function or to compensate for poor function.

Chapter 9: Drooling, continued

Chapter 5 describes in detail treatment techniques which might be appropriate. Chapter 10 lists short-term goals and treatment objectives. Depending on the problem areas noted on the child's oral-motor and swallowing evaluation, you might address the following goals. The treatment objectives that seem most appropriate are listed after the goal:

- Positioning (P) — Child will be positioned appropriately for feeding to allow for optimal intake of food/liquid. (Treatment objectives 2-4, 7, 8)

- Lip Retraction (LR) — Child's oral-motor skills will be enhanced by reducing lip retraction to allow for more efficient eating. (Treatment objectives 1-5)

- Jaw Instability (JI) — Child's oral-motor skills will be enhanced by reducing jaw instability to allow for more efficient eating. (Treatment objectives 1-5)

- Tongue Thrust (TT) — Child's oral-motor skills will be enhanced by reducing tongue thrust to allow for more efficient eating. (Treatment objectives 1-4)

- Low Tone Cheeks (LTC) — Child's oral-motor skills will be enhanced by increasing tone in the cheeks to allow for more efficient eating. (Treatment objectives 1-2)

- Limited Tongue Movement (LT) — Child's oral-motor skills will be enhanced by increasing tongue movement to allow for more efficient eating. (Treatment objectives 1-4)

- Limited Upper Lip Movement (LUL) — Child's oral-motor skills will be enhanced by increasing upper lip movement to allow for more efficient eating. (Treatment objectives 1-7)

- Safety and Efficiency (SE) — Child's eating will be more efficient and safe. (Treatment objectives 1-7)

Behavioral Treatment Approach

If a child has underlying oral-motor deficits or postural difficulties, a behavioral program will not be successful. The underlying physiological problem needs to be addressed first. When the child reaches the point that he is able to hold his head at midline, keep his lips closed, swallow, and have a concept of *wet* and *dry*, it may be appropriate to begin a behavioral program designed to get him to keep his head at midline, keep his lips closed, and swallow more often to decrease the drooling. If decreasing or eliminating the drooling is not a viable

Chapter 9: Drooling, *continued*

goal, then an alternative is to make the child responsible for keeping his face dry by wiping his face with a cloth.

Chapter 8 provides in-depth information about techniques that can be used to reinforce or extinguish a behavior. Those principles are useful when implementing a behavioral program to eliminate drooling. All individuals in the child's daily life need to agree to the goals of such a behavioral program and need to be willing to consistently administer the program.

Chapter 9: Drooling, continued

Appendix 9-A

Questionnaire for Children with Severe Drooling

Client: _____   Date of Evaluation: _____

1. Is drooling constant? _____ yes   _____ no
   If *no*, when does drooling occur most often? _____

2. Does the child seem aware of or uncomfortable with a wet face?
   _____ yes   _____ no

3. Has the drooling been treated in the past? _____ yes   _____ no
   If *yes*, what approaches have been used? _____
   Were they successful? _____ yes   _____ no
   If *yes*, please describe the results. _____
   _____

4. Is the child a mouth-breather? _____ yes   _____ no

5. List any medications the child takes. _____

6. What is the child's reported cognitive level? _____

7. Can the child follow one-step directions? _____ yes   _____ no
   two-step directions? _____ yes   _____ no

8. Does the child understand the concepts of *wet/dry*? _____ yes   _____ no

9. Does the child keep hands in the mouth? _____ yes   _____ no

10. Describe the caregiver's concerns about the drooling. _____
    _____

11. Does the child have any dental problems? (Please describe.) _____
    _____
    If so, has the child seen a dentist? _____ yes   _____ no
    If *yes*, please explain. _____

Chapter 9: Drooling, *continued*

References

Brodsky, L. "Drooling in Children. Pediatric Swallowing and Feeding." In Arvedson, J.C. and Brodsky, L. (eds.) *Pediatric Swallowing and Feeding: Assessment and Management*, San Diego: Singular Publishing Group, Inc., 1993.

Camp-Bruno, J.A. et al. "Efficacy of Benztropine for Drooling." *Developmental Medicine in Child Neurology*, Vol. 31, 1989, pp. 309-319.

Crysdale, W.S. and White, A. "Sub-Mandibular Duct Relocation for Drooling: A Ten-Year Experience with 194 Patients." *Otolaryngology — Head and Neck Surgery*, Vol. 101, 1989, pp. 87-92.

Crysdale, W.S. et al. "The Drooling Patient: Team Evaluation and Management. "*International Journal of Pediatric Otorhinolaryngology*, Vol. 9, 1985, pp. 241-248.

Johnson, H. and Scott, A. *A Practical Approach to Saliva Control*. San Antonio: Communication Skill Builders, a division of The Psychological Corporation, 1993, pp. 20-28.

Limbrock, G.J. et al. "Chewing and Swallowing Dysfunctions in Children with Cerebral Palsy: Treatment According to Castillo-Morales." *Journal of Dentistry for Children*, Nov./Dec. 1990, pp. 445-451.

Chapter 10: Goals and Treatment Objectives

When establishing a treatment plan, select long-term and short-term goals and treatment objectives. The long-term goal(s) should reflect where you think the child will be at the end of treatment. Short-term goals are chosen as targets for a shorter period of time, such as several months. Short-term goals are written in functional terms (i.e., they should describe what the child will be able to do in day-to-day situations). They should be written in terms that payers, consumers, and others who are not SLPs can understand.

To document progress over shorter durations (e.g., monthly summary), the short-term goal must be broken into smaller steps. These smaller steps are called *treatment objectives*. Treatment objectives can be written so that they are measurable over a short period of time. Each treatment objective listed below can be modified to include a variety of information (e.g., a percentage of time the activity will occur, a number of times you expect that response from the child, a length of time you expect the child to maintain a position, a certain situation in which you want the behavior to occur). Because you will probably choose one or more of these variables to measure the child's progress, the treatment objectives below do not contain percentages, times, places, etc. Make these additions to the treatment objectives you choose for each child.

The treatment objectives for the short-term goals related to behavioral feeding disorders (e.g., Readiness and Aversion [RA], Foods Tolerated [FT], Intake Amount [IA], and Appropriate Environment [AE]) are particularly suited to breaking into smaller steps. For example, *Foods Tolerated* contains three treatment objectives designed to increase the number of flavors, textures, and temperatures the child will swallow. Using only treatment objective FT-1, you can see how this can be broken down into many smaller, more measurable steps.

First modify the concept of "swallow" to a series of simpler actions to be accomplished in sequence:

FT-1(a) Child will touch lips with spoon with banana flavor in 1/8 teaspoon amount on ____ consecutive trials without exhibiting negative behaviors.

FT-1(b) Child will touch tongue with spoon with banana flavor in 1/8 teaspoon amount on ____ consecutive trials without exhibiting negative behaviors.

FT-1(c) Child will place spoon with 1/8 teaspoon banana flavor in mouth on ____ consecutive trials without exhibiting negative behaviors.

FT-1(d) Child will clear spoon of 1/8 teaspoon of banana flavor and swallow on ____ consecutive trials without exhibiting negative behaviors.

Chapter 10: Goals and Treatment Objectives, continued

Next vary the amount you expect the child to swallow:

FT-1(e)   Child will clear spoon of 1/4 teaspoon of banana flavor and swallow on ____ consecutive trials without exhibiting negative behaviors.

FT-1(f)   Child will clear spoon of 1/2 teaspoon of banana flavor and swallow on ____ consecutive trials without exhibiting negative behaviors.

You can also gradually increase the number of consecutive trials targeted without negative behaviors and can also define which negative behaviors you want to extinguish (e.g., throwing spoon after taking bite, spitting food out, vomiting). There are endless combinations possible to allow you write treatment objectives precise enough to reflect the changes that often take place in very small steps.

Because we are working with children, most of the treatment objectives are written in passive terms (i.e., what will happen to the child) rather than describing the active response you will get from the child (e.g., "Child will be positioned prone with hand under jaw for support."). Other treatment objectives are written to describe the behavioral response you want to elicit from the child (e.g., "Child will show reduced sensitivity during eating using head flexion.").

You will likely need to choose more than one short-term goal and might choose one or more treatment objectives for each short-term goal. A specific treatment objective may occur for more than one short-term goal (e.g., the treatment objective "Child will demonstrate increased tongue stability and forward movement as a result of tapping under chin on base of tongue" appears as a treatment objective for bunchy tongue and tongue retraction).

Long-Term Goals

1. Infant/child will maintain adequate nutrition and hydration by mouth.

2. Infant/child will consume a diet of foods and liquids typical for developmental peers without complications.

3. Infant/child will maintain adequate nutrition and hydration via alternative means.

4. Infant/child's caregiver will demonstrate understanding of safe feeding techniques.

5. Infant/child's abnormal/immature oral-motor patterns and movements will decrease.

Chapter 10: Goals and Treatment Objectives, *continued*

Short-Term Goals

The following short-term goals each have treatment objectives. The short-term goal is given an abbreviation (e.g., JI for Jaw Instability) and the treatment objectives are numbered using that abbreviation (e.g., JI-1, JI-2).

Master List of Short-Term Goals

State Alert (SA)	Tongue Retraction (TR)
State Calm (SC)	Limited Tongue Movement (LT)
Positioning (P)	Limited Upper Lip Movement (LUL)
Weak Suck (WS)	Hyperactive Gag (HG)
Suck-Swallow-Breathe (SSB)	Aspiration (A)
Jaw Thrust (JT)	Safety and Efficiency (SE)
Jaw Retraction (JR)	Readiness and Aversion (RA)
Lip Retraction (LR)	Food Tolerance (FT)
Jaw Clench (JC)	Intake Amount (IA)
Jaw Instability (JI)	Appropriate Eating (AE)
Tongue Thrust (TT)	Oral Stimulation of Non-Oral Feeder (OSNO)
Bunchy Tongue (BT)	
Low Tone Cheeks (LTC)	Drooling (DR)
Tonic Bite Reflex (TBR)	Gastroesophageal Reflux Disease (GERD)
Oral Hypersensitivty (OH)	

Short-Term Goal: State Alert (SA)

Child will achieve appropriate state of alertness/attention before feeding interaction begins to allow for an optimal feeding experience.

Treatment Objectives

SA-1   Child will be alerted through movement/touch using texture, warm/cold stimuli, massage to palms and soles of feet, rocking side to side, light tickles, vibration, and/or elicitation of rooting.

SA-2   Child will be alerted through taste/smell using foods with sharp tastes, herbs and spices, and/or strong/unique smells.

SA-3   Child will be alerted through visual input using bright colors, shiny objects, moving objects, movement in peripheral vision, and/or contrast of color and shape.

SA-4   Child will be alerted through auditory input using unexpected or loud noises and/or speech with varying volumes, pitches, and rhythm.

Chapter 10: Goals and Treatment Objectives, *continued*

Short-Term Goal: State Calm (SC)

Child will achieve appropriate calm state before feeding interaction begins and will return to a calm state during feeding if signs of distress are demonstrated to allow optimal feeding experience.

Treatment Objectives

SC-1   Child will be calmed through movement/touch using stable position, swaddling, slow rocking or bouncing, establishing non-nutritive sucking, using heavier utensils, foods with more texture, and/or deep pressure to limbs and trunk.

SC-2   Child will be calmed through taste/smell using bland foods.

SC-3   Child will be calmed through visual input using neutral colors, dull objects, and/or no moving objects.

SC-4   Child will be calmed through auditory input using soft, repetitive sounds, music with slow tempo and regular rhythm, and/or white noise.

Short-Term Goal: Positioning (P)

Child will be positioned appropriately for feeding to allow optimal intake of food/liquid.

Treatment Objectives

P-1   Child will be held/placed in semi-reclined position.

P-2   Child will be positioned seated beside the feeder with support provided.

P-3   Child will be positioned upright with feet, hips, and knees at 90°.

P-4   Child will be positioned with neck elongation and chin tuck.

P-5   Child will be positioned in sidelying position.

P-6   Child will be positioned in a prone position.

P-7   Child's hypertonicity will be inhibited before positioning.

P-8   Child will be stimulated for increased muscle tone to compensate for hypotonicity before positioning.

Chapter 10: Goals and Treatment Objectives, *continued*

Short-Term Goal: Weak Suck (WS)

Child's strength and coordination of suck will be enhanced to allow for more efficient eating.

Treatment Objectives

WS-1   Child will achieve better posture during bottle feeding with elongation of neck and/or slight neck flexion.

WS-2   Child will be given jaw and cheek support during sucking.

WS-3   Child will be given heightened stimulation through negative pressure on the nipple, firm pressure to the palate, lingual stroking/tapping to increase tone, and/or firm pressure on the tongue from the nipple.

Short-Term Goal: Suck-Swallow-Breathe (SSB)

Child's coordination of suck-swallow-breathe will be improved to allow for more efficient eating.

Treatment Objectives

SSB-1   Child will be provided with external pacing by removing nipple from the mouth and/or tilting the bottle down to stop flow of liquid.

SSB-2   Child will be provided slower flow of liquid by using slower flow nipple and/or by thickening fluids.

SSB-3   Child will practice coordinating suck-swallow-breathe using non-nutritive sucking.

Short-Term Goal: Jaw Thrust (JT)

Child's oral-motor skills will be enhanced by eliminating jaw thrust to allow for more efficient eating.

Treatment Objectives

JT-1   Child will achieve better sitting posture with trunk and pelvis aligned, shoulders forward, neck elongated, and chin tucked.

JT-2   Child will be presented with a calm environment during treatment.

JT-3   Child will be positioned prone with hand under jaw for support.

The Source for Pediatric Dysphagia

Chapter 10: Goals and Treatment Objectives, continued

JT-4   Child's hypersensitive reaction to contact with teeth will be reduced through firm pressure to face, gums, and teeth.

JT-5   Child's hypersensitive reaction to contact with teeth will be minimized by providing support for jaw closure to increase stability.

JT-6   Child will experience increased sensory input to the tongue through exploration of toys and/or toothbrushing.

JT-7   Child will increase ability to maintain jaw closure by holding objects between teeth.

JT-8   Child will be provided jaw support during eating.

Short-Term Goal: Jaw Retraction (JR)

Child's oral-motor skills will be enhanced by reducing jaw retraction to allow for more efficient eating.

Treatment Objectives

JR-1   Child will achieve better sitting posture with trunk and pelvis aligned, shoulders forward, neck elongated, and chin tucked.

JR-2   Child will be presented with a calm environment during treatment.

JR-3   Child will be positioned prone with hand under jaw for support.

Short-Term Goal: Lip Retraction (LR)

Child's oral-motor skills will be enhanced by reducing lip retraction to allow for more efficient eating.

Treatment Objectives

LR-1   Child will achieve better sitting posture with trunk and pelvis aligned, shoulders forward, neck elongated, and chin tucked.

LR-2   Child will be presented with a calm environment during treatment.

LR-3   Child's cheeks will be vibrated between middle and index finger to promote lip closure.

LR-4   Child's face will be vibrated from nose down through upper lip to promote lip closure.

LR-5   Child's face will be molded with washcloth to stimulate lip closure.

Chapter 10: Goals and Treatment Objectives, continued

Short-Term Goal: Jaw Clench (JC)

Child's oral-motor skills will be enhanced by eliminating jaw clench to allow for more efficient eating.

Treatment Objectives

JC-1   Child will achieve better sitting posture with trunk and pelvis aligned, shoulders forward, neck elongated, and chin tucked.

JC-2   Child will be presented with a calm environment during treatment.

JC-3   Child will be positioned prone with hand under jaw for support.

JC-4   Child's hypersensitive reaction to contact with teeth will be reduced through firm pressure to face, gums, and teeth.

JC-5   Child's hypersensitive reaction to contact with teeth will be minimized by providing support for jaw closure to increase stability.

JC-6   Child will experience increased sensory input to the tongue through exploration of toys and/or toothbrushing.

Short-Term Goal: Jaw Instability (JI)

Child's oral-motor skills will be enhanced by reducing jaw instability to allow for more efficient eating.

Treatment Objectives

JI-1   Child will achieve better sitting posture with trunk and pelvis aligned, shoulders forward, neck elongated, and chin tucked.

JI-2   Child will increase ability to maintain jaw closure by holding objects between teeth.

JI-3   Child will be provided jaw support during eating.

JI-4   Child's jaw muscles will receive increased tactile and proprioceptive stimulation through rhythmic tapping on cheeks and TMJ.

JI-5   Child will increase ability to achieve jaw closure after quick stretch of the masseter.

Chapter 10: Goals and Treatment Objectives, continued

Short-Term Goal: Tongue Thrust (TT)

Child's oral-motor skills will be enhanced by reducing tongue thrust to allow for more efficient eating.

Treatment Objectives

TT-1   Child will achieve better sitting posture with trunk and pelvis aligned, shoulders forward, neck elongated, and chin tucked.

TT-2   Child will be provided with jaw support during eating.

TT-3   Child will develop more mature tongue movement through exposure to textured foods.

TT-4   Child will develop tongue bowl response through even pressure applied by spoon and/or vibration of tongue.

Short-Term Goal: Bunchy Tongue (BT)

Child's oral-motor skills will be enhanced by reducing bunchy tongue to allow for more efficient eating.

Treatment Objectives

BT-1   Child will experience increased sensory input to the tongue through exploration of toys and/or toothbrushing.

BT-2   Child will receive heightened sensory input to the tongue through vibration.

BT-3   Child will demonstrate increased tongue stability and forward movement when using chin-tuck position.

BT-4   Child will demonstrate increased tongue stability and forward movement as a result of tapping under chin on base of tongue.

BT-5   Child will achieve more relaxed tongue during non-nutritive sucking following lingual stroking/tapping to flatten tongue.

Short-Term Goal: Low Tone Cheeks (LTC)

Child's oral-motor skills will be enhanced by increasing tone in the cheeks to allow for more efficient eating.

Chapter 10: Goals and Treatment Objectives, continued

Treatment Objectives

LTC-1 Child will demonstrate increased tone of jaw muscles as a result of tactile and proprioceptive stimulation through rhythmic tapping on cheeks and TMJ.

LTC-2 Child will improve ability to suck from a straw when using squeeze bottle with straw and/or placing a small portion of straw in mouth.

Short-Term Goal: Tonic Bite Reflex (TBR)

Child's oral-motor skills will be enhanced by reducing tonic bite reflex to allow for more efficient eating.

Treatment Objectives

TBR-1 Child will achieve better sitting posture with trunk and pelvis aligned, shoulders forward, neck elongated, and chin tucked.

TBR-2 Child's hypersensitive reaction to contact with teeth will be reduced through firm pressure to face, gums, and teeth.

TBR-3 Child's hypersensitive reaction to contact with teeth will be minimized by providing support for jaw closure to increase stability.

TBR-4 Child will experience increased sensory input to the tongue through exploration of toys and/or toothbrushing.

Short-Term Goal: Oral Hypersensitivity (OH)

Child's oral-motor skills will be enhanced by reducing oral hypersensitivity to allow for more efficient eating.

Treatment Objectives

OH-1 Child will tolerate graded stimulation to trunk, neck, face, and mouth.

OH-2 Child's hypersensitive reaction to contact with teeth will be reduced through firm pressure to face, gums, and teeth.

OH-3 Child's hypersensitive reaction to contact with teeth will be minimized by providing support for jaw closure to increase stability.

OH-4 Child will experience increased sensory input to the tongue through exploration of toys and/or toothbrushing.

Chapter 10: Goals and Treatment Objectives, continued

OH-5   Child will increase tolerance of stimulation in the oral cavity from vibration.

OH-6   Child will show reduced sensitivity to stimulation on the tongue through "tongue walking" posteriorly with tongue blade.

OH-7   Child will show reduced sensitivity during eating by using head flexion.

Short-Term Goal: Tongue Retraction (TR)

Child's oral-motor skills will be enhanced by reducing tongue retraction to allow for more efficient eating.

Treatment Objectives

TR-1   Child will be positioned prone with hand under jaw for support.

TR-2   Child will demonstrate increased tongue stability and forward movement when using chin-tuck position.

TR-3   Child will demonstrate increased tongue stability and forward movement as a result of tapping under chin on base of tongue.

TR-4   Child's tongue will flatten in response to quick lateral vibrations on center of tongue, non-nutritive sucking and/or lingual stroking/tapping.

Short-Term Goal: Limited Tongue Movement (LT)

Child's oral-motor skills will be enhanced by increasing tongue movement to allow for more efficient eating.

Treatment Objectives

LT-1   Child will increase tolerance of stimulation in the oral cavity from vibration.

LT-2   Child will demonstrate increased tongue stability and forward movement when using chin-tuck position.

LT-3   Child will demonstrate increased tongue stability and forward movement as a result of tapping under chin on base of tongue.

LT-4   Child's tongue will flatten in response to quick lateral vibrations on center of tongue.

Chapter 10: Goals and Treatment Objectives, *continued*

Short-Term Goal: Limited Upper Lip Movement (LUL)

Child's oral-motor skills will be enhanced by increasing upper lip movement to allow for more efficient eating.

Treatment Objectives

LUL-1   Child's cheeks will be vibrated between middle and index finger to promote lip closure.

LUL-2   Child's face will be vibrated from nose down through upper lip to promote lip closure.

LUL-3   Child will demonstrate increased tone in the jaw muscles as a result of tactile and proprioceptive stimulation through rhythmic tapping on cheeks and TMJ.

LUL-4   Child will demonstrate upper lip movement as a result of vibration of upper lip.

LUL-5   Child will demonstrate upper lip movement as a result of quick stretch.

LUL-6   Child will demonstrate upper lip movement as a result of sensory input to lip from toys and/or tastes.

LUL-7   Child will improve ability to suck from a straw when using squeeze bottle with straw and/or placing a small portion of straw in mouth.

Short-Term Goal: Hyperactive Gag (HG)

Child's tolerance of oral-motor stimulation and eating will increase by eliminating hyperactive gag.

Treatment Objectives

HG-1   Child's hypersensitive reaction to contact with teeth will be reduced through firm pressure to face, gums, and teeth.

HG-2   Child's hypersensitive reaction to contact with teeth will be minimized by providing support for jaw closure to increase stability.

HG-3   Child will experience increased sensory input to the tongue through exploration of toys and/or toothbrushing.

HG-4   Child will increase tolerance of stimulation in the oral cavity from vibration.

Chapter 10: Goals and Treatment Objectives, continued

HG-5   Child will show reduced sensitivity to stimulation on the tongue through "tongue walking" posteriorly with tongue blade.

Short-Term Goal: Aspiration (A)

Child will swallow more safely because of reduced risk of aspiration.

Treatment Objectives

A-1   Speed of initiation of pharyngeal swallow will be increased through sucking cold pacifier and/or use of sour bolus.

A-2   Size of the bolus will be reduced so that bolus does not enter airway during delay.

A-3   Greater airway protection will be provided during the swallow through slight chin-tuck posture, thickened feedings, and/or slower flow rate.

A-4   Pharyngeal residue will be reduced after the swallow through multiple swallows and/or use of liquid wash.

Short-Term Goal: Safety and Efficiency (SE)

Child's eating will be more efficient and safe.

Treatment Objectives

SE-1   Child will be presented with _____ liquids from spoon, cut-out cup, and/or sunken lid cup.

SE-2   When presented with _____ liquids, child will be given jaw support and/or lip support.

SE-3   Child will be presented with smooth textures from _____ spoon.

SE-4   When presented with food on spoon, child will be assisted with jaw support, support for lip closure, and/or downward pressure on spoon on tongue.

SE-5   Child will be presented with liquids from regular straw, straw in squeeze bottle, thick-walled tubing, and/or straw dipped into liquid.

SE-6   Child will be presented with foods that have to be masticated on lateral chewing surfaces and/or on midline of tongue.

SE-7   When child is presented foods that have to be masticated, child will be assisted with jaw support and/or lip support.

Chapter 10: Goals and Treatment Objectives, continued

> *Note: Short-term goals* Readiness and Aversion (RA), Foods Tolerated (FT), Intake Amount (IA), *and* Appropriate Eating (AE) *are designed for behavioral feeding disorders. However, as described in Chapter 8, there is often a physiological component to behavioral feeding disorders. Thus you may also choose short-term goals and treatment objectives to improve function depending on the child's deficit areas. Many children with behavioral feeding disorders will also exhibit oral hypersensitivity and hyperactive gag, so short-term goals* OH *and* HG *may often be selected along with one or more of the goals listed below. The* Oral Stimulation of Non-Oral Feeder (OSNO) *goal is grouped with behavioral feeding as a preventative goal. If children who are totally non-oral are not provided with appropriate stimulation, they are more likely to develop behavioral feeding disorders when later introduced to PO intake.*

Short-Term Goal: Readiness and Aversion (RA)

Child will increase readiness for and decrease aversion to oral feeding.

Treatment Objectives

RA-1   Child will play with utensils and place them in mouth with no food present.

RA-2   Child will sit in chair for increasing periods of time.

RA-3   Child will participate in non-feeding activities while seated at the table.

RA-4   Child will follow simple directions without oppositional behavior.

Short-Term Goal: Food Tolerance (FT)

Child will increase the number and types of foods tolerated.

Treatment Objectives

FT-1   Child will swallow _____ flavor in _____ amount without exhibiting negative behaviors.

FT-2   Child will swallow _____ texture in _____ amount without exhibiting negative behaviors.

FT-3   Child will swallow _____ temperature in _____ amount without exhibiting negative behaviors.

Chapter 10: Goals and Treatment Objectives, *continued*

Short-Term Goal: Intake Amount (IA)

Child will increase the amount of food/liquid taken by mouth while decreasing amount given by tube.

Treatment Objectives

IA-1   Child will be presented with oral feedings at regularly scheduled feeding times prior to being given any tube feeding.

IA-2   The amount of tube feeding presented will be reduced at the tube feeding immediately prior to the meal at which oral food will be given.

IA-3   Tube feeding will be diluted (consult with dietitian or physician) to increase feeling of hunger.

Short-Term Goal: Appropriate Eating (AE)

Child will generalize appropriate eating skills to other environments.

Treatment Objectives

AE-1   Caregivers will be introduced into the feeding therapy session as observers.

AE-2   Caregivers will participate in the feeding therapy session.

AE-3   Caregivers will institute behavioral feeding program in more natural settings.

Short-Term Goal: Oral Stimulation of Non-Oral Feeder (OSNO)

Child who is fed non-orally will be provided pleasurable oral/facial stimulation.

Treatment Objectives

OSNO-1   Child will be held during non-oral feeding.

OSNO-2   Child will be presented with pacifier/finger to suck during non-oral feeding.

OSNO-3   Child will be presented with smells and tastes during non-oral feedings.

Chapter 10: Goals and Treatment Objectives, *continued*

> *Note: As noted in Chapter 9, there are many other short-term goals that may need to be addressed to control drooling before working on the following objectives which are designed to have the child take more responsibility for maintaining a dry face. There are also treatment objectives to compensate for decreased function.*
>
> *Depending on the needs of the child, you may want to consider the following to actually increase function: Positioning 2-4, 7, and 8; Lip Retraction 1-5; Limited Upper Lip Movement 1-7; Jaw Retraction 1-3; Jaw Instability 1-5; Limited Tongue Movement 1-4; Safe and Efficient Swallow 1-7.*

Short-Term Goal: Drooling (DR)

Child will decrease drooling and increase amount of time face is dry.

Treatment Objectives

DR-1   Child will lift head to upright and midline consistently when given cues.

DR-2   Child will maintain head at upright/midline.

DR-3   Child will close lips consistently when given cues.

DR-4   Child will maintain lip closure.

DR-5   Child will swallow saliva when cued.

DR-6   Child will swallow saliva without cues.

DR-7   Child will wipe face consistently when given cues.

DR-8   Child will wipe face independently.

Chapter 10: Goals and Treatment Objectives, continued

> *Note: As discussed in Chapter 2, GERD can be treated behaviorally, medically, or surgically. The SLP is often involved in carrying out the behavioral objectives and that is why suggested objectives are listed here. Close consultation with the child's physician is necessary when determining which, if any, of these objectives might be appropriate for a particular child.*

Short-Term Goal: Gastroesophageal Reflux Disease (GERD)

Child will exhibit a reduction in symptoms of gastroesophageal reflux (e.g., less irritability).

Treatment Objectives

GERD-1   Child will be held upright during feeding.

GERD-2   Child will be given smaller amounts at more frequent feedings.

GERD-3   Child's formula will be thickened.

GERD-4   Child will be positioned prone and on incline after feeding.

Chapter 11: Tools for Feeding

Infants and children with feeding disorders often require specialized seating and feeding utensils. Consult with a physical therapist when selecting a seating device. Provide input on what you believe the child is able to achieve for self-feeding (e.g., Is the child ready to sit and eat finger foods?). Also provide input on the type of support needed for appropriate positioning for feeding (e.g., Can the child hold his head up or does he need support? Does the child need to be in a flexed position?).

The information provided on pages 241-248 has been summarized from a variety of sources. The addresses were confirmed to the best extent possible. Many of these tools and utensils are available in children's departments of department stores or discount stores like Sears™, Wal-Mart®, Super Target®, and Toys R Us®.

Chapter 11: Tools for Feeding, *continued*

Seating Devices

Only children with mild problems in head and trunk control can be seated in a standard seating system like the Tumble Forms® Feeder Seat.		Sammons Preston, Inc. P.O. Box 5071 Bolingbrook, IL 60440-5071 Phone: 1-800-323-5547 Fax: 1-800-547-4333
Children with more moderate deficits will need seating devices like the Snug Seat® that allow for multiple adjustments.		Snug Seat P.O. Box 1739 Matthews, NC 28106 Phone: 1-800-336-7684 Fax: 704-882-0751
Children with severe deficits in head and trunk control and with severe asymmetry will need a custom-made seating system. These usually involve making a mold of the child's body.	System depends on child's needs.	Most medical supply stores work with companies who make custom molds. See your local dealer.
For use during videofluoroscopic evaluations, you can use a Tumble Forms® seat placed in either the MAMA® Chair or the Hausted® Chair. The Hausted® Chair can be used for older children. For children under 60 lbs., some hospitals use the MAMA Chair. Both have hip, chest, and head restraints.	MAMA® Hausted®	MAMA® Chair and Hausted® Videofluoroscopic Imaging Chair are usually only used in hospitals.
If children need to be fed prone, use a wedge for smaller children or a prone stander for older children.		Sammons Preston, Inc. (see address above)

The Source for Pediatric Dysphagia

Chapter 11: Tools for Feeding, continued

Pacifiers

Mini MAM® Orthodontic Newborn Pacifier can be used with newborns and premature infants.		Mini-MAM®, The First Years®, NUK®, and Playtex® pacifiers can be found in most discount department stores.
First Years® Kip Orthodontic Pacifier helps establish a normal tongue position during sucking.		
NUK® Orthodontic Pacifier can be used with infants up to about 18 months of age.		NUK® pacifiers can also be purchased by contacting: New Visions Attn: Mealtimes Catalog Route 1, Box 175-S Faber, VA 22938 Phone: 804-361-2285 Fax: 804-361-1807
Playtex® Pacifier is shaped like the Playtex Nurser®, but infants with reduced oral-motor skills have a hard time latching on.		

Chapter 11: Tools for Feeding, *continued*

Nipples

Standard nipples vary in firmness of material and size of hole. Some may have cross cuts in the nipple.		Standard nipples, cross-cut nipples, NUK® nipples, and Playtex® nipples can be found at most discount department stores.
NUK® nipples have an orthodontic shape to fit the mouth.		
Playtex® nipples are short and firm and give a broad base of contact to the lips. Infants with feeding problems characterized by tongue retraction may not be able to latch on.		
Ross Twist-On® nipples are mainly used in hospitals. They are disposable and meant for one-time use only.		Ross Products Division of Abbott Labs 1-800-FORMULA (367-6852)
Preemie nipples are usually made of a softer material with a cross cut. Softer nipples work well for infants with a weak suck.		Mead Johnson Nutritionals Phone: 1-800-BABY123 (222-9123)

The Source for Pediatric Dysphagia

Chapter 11: Tools for Feeding, continued

Bottles

Standard bottles typically hold 8 ounces (240cc). Juice bottles are smaller than standard bottles and hold 4 ounces (120 cc). Playtex Nursers® have a plastic bag inside a hard plastic shell. The plastic bags create a vacuum as the infant sucks so that the child can be upright or prone and still get liquid. You can also provide slight pressure to the bag for infants with a weak suck.		Standard bottles, juice bottles, angle-neck bottles, and Playtex® Nursers can be found at most discount department stores.
Volu-feed® bottles are often used in the NICU. They hold 2 ounces. They are easier to hold in one hand so you can use that same hand to provide cheek and/or lip support.		Ross Products Division of Abbott Labs 1-800-FORMULA (367-6852)
Angle-neck bottles allow the infant to keep the neck in slight flexion while sucking. They are also good for infants fed in sidelying or prone positions.		New Visions Attn: Mealtimes Catalog Route 1, Box 175-S Faber, VA 22938 Phone: 804-361-2285 Fax: 804-361-1807
Mead Johnson Cleft Palate Nurser® is made of soft plastic so it can be squeezed to help the flow. You can use different nipples on the bottle.		Mead Johnson Nutritionals Phone: 1-800-BABY123 (222-9123)
Haberman Feeders® have a one-way valve in the mouthpiece to allow easy flow of liquid and prevent backflow into the bottle. The nipple is filled before you start feeding. You can change the rate of flow. This bottle is particularly helpful with babies with cleft palates.		Medela, Inc. P.O. Box 660 McHenry, IL 60051 Phone: 1-800-435-8316 Fax: 1-800-995-7867 Or New Visions (see address above)

The Source for Pediatric Dysphagia Copyright © 1998 LinguiSystems, Inc.

Chapter 11: Tools for Feeding, *continued*

Cups

Solo® clear plastic cups have a wide mouth so the child can tip the cup up without tipping the head back. The clear sides let you see how much the child is drinking and also allows you to observe lip function.		Most grocery stores
Tumblemates® cups have a free-flow sipper top.		Tumblemates® cups, Spill Proof® cups, Tommee Tippee® cups, and the MagMag® Training Cup System can be found at most discount department stores.
Spill Proof® cups have a valve with a spring which requires a stronger suck. It also has a slower flow.		
Tommee Tippee® Training Cups have a rounded weighted bottom. They have a spouted lid or sunken lid with small holes. Using the spout perpetuates the sucking pattern rather than moving the child to a more mature swallowing pattern.		
MagMag® Training Cup System can first be fitted with a nipple, then a spout, then a straw, and then a lid.		MagMag® Training Cup System can also be purchased by contacting: Equipment Shop P.O. Box 33 Bedford, MA 01730 Phone: 1-800-525-7681 Fax: 617-275-4094

continued

Chapter 11: Tools for Feeding, *continued*

Cups, *continued*

Infa-Trainer® Cup is made of clear plastic in a tall shape like a bottle which makes it easy for the child to hold. The lid can be turned to adjust the flow of liquid.		New Visions Attn: Mealtimes Catalog Route 1, Box 175-S Faber, VA 22938 Phone: 804-361-2285 Fax: 804-361-1807
Nosey Cups® allow the child to tip the cup up without tipping his head back.		Sammons Preston, Inc. P.O. Box 5071 Bolingbrook, IL 60440-5071 Phone: 1-800-323-5547 Fax: 1-800-547-4333 Smith & Nephew, Inc. P.O. Box 1005 Germantown, WI 53022-8205 Phone: 1-800-558-8633 Fax: 1-800-545-7758

Chapter 11: Tools for Feeding, *continued*

Spoons

Maroon Spoons® are nonbreakable and have flatter bowls than most spoons.		New Visions Attn: Mealtimes Catalog Route 1, Box 175-S Faber, VA 22938 Phone: 804-361-2285 Fax: 804-361-1807 Equipment Shop P.O. Box 33 Bedford, MA 01730 Phone: 1-800-525-7681 Fax: 617-275-4094
Easy Grip® spoons are a good fit for a child's hand, but not for an adult's. Soft Bite® spoons are plastic coated and have small bowls for a good fit in the mouth.		Easy Grip® spoons and Soft Bite spoons can be found at most discount department stores.
Swivel spoons compensate for a child's lack of ability to control the wrist. They can scoop the food and as the child brings it toward his mouth, the bowl swivels so the food doesn't spill.		Sammons Preston, Inc. P.O. Box 5071 Bolingbrook, IL 60440-5071 Phone: 1-800-323-5547 Fax: 1-800-547-4333

Chapter 11: Tools for Feeding, *continued*

Other Utensils and Tools

Scooper bowls and plates have raised rims to scoop against. They have suction cups on the bottom to keep the bowls/plates from moving away from the child. Plate guards or food guards can be affixed to a regular plate. They provide the same function as the scooper plate.	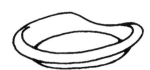 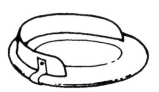	Sammons Preston, Inc. P.O. Box 5071 Bolingbrook, IL 60440-5071 Phone: 1-800-323-5547 Fax: 1-800-547-4333 Smith & Nephew, Inc. P.O. Box 1005 Germantown, WI 53022-8205 Phone: 1-800-558-8633 Fax: 1-800-545-7758
NUK® Toothbrush Trainer Sets provide a graded change in the texture of the head of the brush.	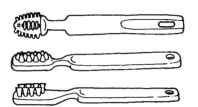	New Visions Attn: Mealtimes Catalog Route 1, Box 175-S Faber, VA 22938 Phone: 804-361-2285 Fax: 804-361-1807 Equipment Shop P.O. Box 33 Bedford, MA 01730 Phone: 1-800-525-7681 Fax: 617-275-4094

Chapter 11: Tools for Feeding, continued

References

Arvedson, J. and Brodsky, L. *Pediatric Swallowing and Feeding Assessment and Management*, San Diego: Singular Publishing Group, Inc., 1993, pp. 271 and 427.

Morris, S.E. and Klein, M.D. *Pre-Feeding Skills*, San Antonio: Communication Skill Builders, a division of The Psychological Corporation, 1987, pp. 356-389.

Rosenthal, S. et al. *Dysphagia and the Child with Developmental Disabilities: Medical, Clinical, and Family Interventions*, San Diego: Singular Publishing Group, Inc., 1995, pp. 197-198.

Wolf, L.F. and Glass, R.P. *Feeding and Swallowing Disorders in Infancy: Assessment and Management*, San Antonio: Therapy Skill Builders, a division of The Psychological Corporation, 1992, pp. 77, 404, 413, 417.

Glossary

acute gastroenteritis — a sudden onset of inflammation of stomach and intestines

ankyloglossia — short frenulum

anomaly — something which deviates from the norm

anterior — in front of (e.g., the heart is anterior to the spine)

anti-cholinergic — designed to dry out secretions

apnea — temporary stopping of breathing

atelectasis — alveoli in lungs don't fully expand or collapse

atresia — absence of normal opening

atresia choanae — posterior cavity of nose is not open

bradycardia — drop in heart rate below 90-100 beats per minute

bronchiolitis — inflammation of the bronchioles (small branches of the lungs)

bronchopulmonary dysplasia — chronic lung disorder often seen in neonates who required a lot of ventilator support

bronchospasm — spasm of bronchial tubes

catabolic — use of body stores/tissues to support energy needs

choane — posterior cavity of the nose

cholestatic jaundice — jaundice caused by accumulation of bile in the liver

Glossary, *continued*

coloboma	developmental anomaly of the eye
contractures	an abnormal shortening and tightening of a muscle
cyanotic	bluish color of skin due to reduced levels of oxygen in the blood
cystic fibrosis	common and often fatal disease of childhood in which an excess amount of mucous causes progressive lung damage
decerebate posturing	extremities are stiff and extended with the head retracted
decorticate	characteristic of a point of lesion at or above the upper brain stem; the point is rigidly still with arms flexed, fists clenched, and legs extended
decorticate/ decerebrate posturing	after severe brain damage, a flexed, almost fetal position
dental caries	cavities in the teeth
distal	farthest from a reference point or farthest from the center (e.g., the part of the esophagus near the entrance to the stomach is considered distal since it is the farthest from the starting point of the esophagus)
diuretics	medicine to stimulate the flow of urine
edema	swelling from an accumulation of fluid
embryogenesis	development of the embryo
emesis	vomiting

Glossary, *continued*

encephalopathy	a general term describing a disorder of the brain; often used when a more specific diagnosis cannot be made
encopresis	incontinence of feces which is not due to a defect or illness
enteral	within or passing through the intestines
enterocolitis	inflammation of small intestine and colon
esophagitis	inflammation of the esophagus
extrapyramidal	set of pathways that connect subcortical motor nuclei
extra-uterine	occuring outside the uterus
fistula	a passage or tract
flexion	opposite of hyperextension; bent
fundus of stomach	part of the stomach to the left of and above the level of the opening between the stomach and the esophagus
gastrostomy	an opening in the stomach
gavage feedings	feeding through a tube
genital hypoplasia	incomplete development of the genitals
glossoplexy	surgically affixing the tip of the tongue to the lower lip
glossoptosis	tongue falling back into the airway
hematemesis	vomiting blood

Glossary, *continued*

hyperextension	excessive straightening of a flexed limb
hypertonic	high tone; increased tone
hypoplasia	incomplete development of tissue or organ
hypotonic	low tone; decreased tone
hypoxic/hypoxia	abnormally low amount of oxygen (e.g., hypoxic brain damage is caused by decreased supply of oxygen to the brain)
inflammatory bowel disease	gastrointestinal disorder caused by inflammation of the intestinal tract
interstitial fibrosis	fibrous tissue that forms in a gap
intestinal malrotation	abnormal twisting of intestines
laryngo-tracheomalacia	softening of the cartilages in the larynx and trachea, causing them to collapse on inhalation
laryngomalacia	softening of the cartilage in the larynx
laryngospasm	spasm of the larynx
lateral	pertaining to the side or situated at the side (e.g., the arm is lateral to the trunk)
mandibular hypoplasia	incomplete development of the mandible
melena	bloody stool
microcephaly	small head size

Glossary, *continued*

micrognathia	abnormally small or abnormally positioned mandible
Moëbius Sequence	sequence of events in utero as child is developing; characterized by damage to cranial nerves which results in weakness in the lower face
mucosal injury	damage to the mucosa that lines a body part (e.g., esophagus)
multiple intestinal atresia	absence of openings throughout the intestines
myelodysplasia	defective development of the spinal cord
necrotizing	cells dying as a result of disease or injury
neonate	newborn infant
NPO	nothing by mouth
oro-tracheal	area of the oral cavity and trachea
osteopenia	decreased bone mass
oxygen saturation	amount of oxygen in the blood, expressed as a % of 100
parasympathetic nervous system	part of the autonomic nervous system responsible for calming the body (e.g., slows the heart rate, increases peristalsis in the intestines, increases salivation)
parenteral	bypassing the digestive system
pericardium	the sac enclosing the heart
peristalsis	progression of contractions and relaxation

Glossary, *continued*

peristaltic wave	muscle contraction and relaxation
phasic bite reflex	present from birth until about 3-5 months of age; a rhythmical opening and closing of the jaw when gums are stimulated
phenylketonuria (PKU)	a metabolic disorder present at birth; if not treated, results in severe mental retardation
Pierre Robin	a cluster of symptoms including small mandible, tongue falling back in mouth, and cleft of hard palate
polyhydramnios	excessive amniotic fluid
posterior	situated behind a part of the body (e.g., the spine is posterior to the heart)
proximal	next to or nearest the point of attachment or origin, a central point
reactive airway disease	any airway disease caused by reaction to an allergen (e.g., asthma)
scapular adduction	shoulder blades pulled toward each other
septic/sepsis	abnormal presence of bacteria
spina bifida	a defect of the skin, spinal column, and spinal cord occurring in utero; the spine pushes out into a membranous sac and the nerves below it are not connected
steroids	medication used to treat swelling and inflammation
strictures	abnormal narrowing of opening or passage
stridor	a harsh sound; often used to describe noisy inhalation

Glossary, *continued*

subglottic stenosis	narrowing of the trachea below the vocal cords
sucking	begins around 6-9 months
suckling	occurs from birth to 6-9 months
supine	lying on the back
surfactant	a substance in the lungs that helps keep the alveoli expanded (partially inflated alveoli makes it easier to breathe)
sustained bite pattern	mature pattern of biting where teeth close easily to bite through food
sympathetic nervous system	part of the autonomic nervous system responsible for alerting the body (e.g., accelerates the heart rate, raises blood pressure, dilates the pupils)
tachycardia	elevated heart rate
tachynpea	elevated level of breathing
toxemia	toxic products in the blood
tracheomalacia	softening of the cartilages in the trachea
transcutaneous arterial oxygen levels	oxygen levels in the blood obtained through sensor placed on the skin
transitional feeding	a stage of eating moving from a liquid to a solid diet
velopharyngeal	related to the velum and pharynx

Dorland's Pocket Medical Dictionary. Philadelphia: W.B. Saunders, 1968.